A Practical Guide to
Sports First Aid

A Practical Guide to
Sports First Aid

Wayne Gill

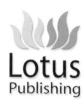

Lotus
Publishing

First published in 2005 by
Lotus Publishing
9 Roman Way, Chichester, PO19 3QN

Author's Note and Disclaimer
I refer to 'he' throughout this book for the sake of grammatical consistency. Whilst the information herein is supplied in good faith, no responsibility is taken by either the publisher or the author for any damage, injury or loss, however caused, which may arise from the use of the information provided.

Acknowledgements
John Sharkey, author of the section on neuromuscular therapy. Dr. Sam Scheinberg, author of the chapter on the SAM® Splint. Gina T. Batt, Seaberg Company liaison officer. Pat Abercromby and Davina Thomson for administration. Thanks also to Magister Consulting Limited for the use of the electrical system of the heart diagram (figure 14.2).

Anatomical Drawings : Amanda Williams
Photographs : Wayne Gill, Noreen Hoban, Damian Spelman
Models : Paul Joyce, John Robinson, Eliseah Robinson
Text and Cover Design : Chris Fulcher
Printed and Bound in the UK by Scotprint

British Library Cataloguing in Publication Data
A CIP record for this book is available from the British Library

ISBN 0 9543188 6 2

Contents

Foreword 7

Introduction 9

Chapter 1   The Basics 11

Chapter 2   Introduction to First Aid 17

Chapter 3   The Circulatory System, Wounds and Bleeding 23

Chapter 4   Basic Life Support 29

Chapter 5   Fractures and the Skeleton 47

Chapter 6   SAM® Splint 65

Chapter 7   Soft Tissue Injuries 73

Chapter 8   Spinal Injuries 83

Chapter 9   Head Injuries 87

Chapter 10   Chest Injuries 93

Chapter 11   Medical Emergencies 97

Chapter 12   Common Minor Sports Injuries 109

Chapter 13   Athletes with Disabilities 115

Chapter 14   BLS and AED 119

Appendix 129

Useful Addresses 141

Index 143

Foreword

There are numerous texts describing the long-term management of chronic problems resulting from trauma of all sorts, and sporting injuries and incidents in particular. While some of these contain descriptions of first aid strategies, few if any summarise all aspects required for the skilled and safe, immediate care of as wide a range of possible injuries and emergencies as this book.

Indeed the book covers far more than trauma. It states explicitly that it has been designed "to teach Sports First Aid Practitioners the essential skills to deal with all medical emergencies they may encounter throughout the sporting industry." This is a wide brief, and the realisation has been superb.

The book however has to be seen as providing reminders and summaries of protocols – in words and pictures – and not as a resource to be used without adequate training. Fortunately, Sports First Aid courses are now widely available, with the specific course for which this book was designed being amongst the best.

No-one working in the field of sport, or rehabilitation, or who is involved in the therapeutic aspects of manual medicine, should be deficient in first aid skills. These are potentially life saving, and when used in less critical settings, potentially career saving.

Outside of competitive sport, it is worth emphasising that, for example, the casual gardener or elderly individual walking in the park is performing physical activity. This has the easy potential for injury that would benefit from skilled first aid, whether the injury resulted from lifting and bending, slipping or stumbling, or some minor deviation from normal patterns of use.

An injury that is well managed at the outset is far more likely to recover fully than one that receives poor or no initial attention. The difference between good and bad (or no) first aid can mean the difference between a rapid return to athletic or other physical activity, compared to a lengthy period of recovery, or no full recovery at all.

Someone once said, "we are all athletes, but only some of us are in training." This can be paraphrased to say we are all capable of offering first aid, but only some of us will do so safely and efficiently.

I for one would not want first aid from someone ill-trained and ignorant of the details of care required for a specific problem, whether a snake bite, a laceration, shock, a heart attack, an obstructed airway, a fracture, dislocation or sprain or any of dozens of other potential emergency situations.

This text is laid out logically, accurately and with a minimum of clutter. It comprises summaries, using bullet points and succinct paragraphs of explanation where needed, as well as clear illustrations. Many people will be grateful for the author's diligence in producing this timely text. It may save lives, and will certainly ease distress and promote recovery.

Leon Chaitow, N. D., D.O.
Senior Lecturer, University of Westminster
Editor, *Journal of Bodywork & Movement Therapies*

Knowing just a little first aid can save a person's life. Everyone should know some first aid. It gives me great pleasure to write a foreword to this book. It is an important publication containing the knowledge, principals, risks and treatments of a wide variety of sports injuries. No stone is left unturned reflecting the competent skills and knowledge of an expert Sports First Aid Practitioner.

This book will be helpful to everyone. A dearth of publications specific to sports first aid presently exist and this publication will fill that void. I found this unique book to be a readable, easy-to-understand and up-to-date account ensuring that the highest standards of sports first aid are administered in a variety of settings for every conceivable scenario. Legal issues, scope of practice, duty of care, check lists, things to do and importantly what not to do are all in this wonderfully crafted text providing the reader with a reference book to refer to time and time again. The scope of this book reflects a breadth of knowledge few others have, yet all of us need.

Diagnosing is exclusively for the medical doctor. However, differential diagnosis within the sports injury scenario can be the difference between life or death. This book provides the reader with the essential knowledge to avoid wasted time adding to pain, discomfort, longer recovery, and missed competitions. The Sports First Aid Practitioner must acquire and develop the skills and knowledge to respond promptly to a wide variety of sports injury scenarios. Issues such as bleeding, wounds, signs and symptoms, life support and when required, bandaging, are just some of the skills demanded to ensure the safe, appropriate and effective treatment of the athlete or indeed a spectator. This book provides that knowledge as a supporting text for any individual participating on a sports first aid course or for practicing and experienced first aid practitioners as a rich and comprehensive text which should be a part of the sports first aid bag at all times. The very nature of participation in sport increases the risk of injury and the Sports First Aid Practitioner is the front line soldier regarding the correct management in the war on injuries.

Immediate and appropriate treatment of an injury is the first step in providing the most effective path to recovery. The Sports First Aid Practitioner must know when to refer an injured athlete to an injury specialist such as a Neuromuscular Therapist (NMT). This text is a historical one providing as it does information on neuromuscular therapy and where athletes can go to find a neuromuscular therapist in their geographical location.

As a member of the Olympic Council of Ireland's medical support team, I am pleased to highly recommend this book to anyone involved in the immediate care of the athlete.

John Sharkey, N.M.T., B.Sc.
OCI Medical Team, Director, National Training Centre, Ireland.

Introduction

The Sports Industry is now so vast that it covers sports that were unheard of up to a few years ago. This increase has given rise to the risk of injuries that affect athletes of all levels and ages. The types of injuries are now so complex, and the sportsman so competitive, that he must return to competition as soon as possible. This course / book will teach therapists injury assessment, remedial exercises, diagnoses and treatment of injuries. Sports therapists who can identify, assess and treat sports injuries are therefore in great demand. It is vital for all clubs and sporting groups to have a qualified skilled Sports First Aid Practitioner at all their training sessions and games. This book has been written to accompany the course for 'The National Qualification in Sports First Aid' (National Training Centre, Ireland).

This course and book have been designed to teach Sports First Aid Practitioners the essential skills required to deal with all medical emergencies that may be encountered throughout the sporting industry. Dealing with pre-hospital trauma is the Sports First Aid Practitioners' responsibility and this course / book will teach them the relevant skills to diagnose and treat injuries to a professional standard while awaiting the support of medical personnel.

1. The Basics

The Good Samaritan Act

The Good Samaritan Act (law) is also known as the Emergency Medical Aid Act in some countries. Sports First Aid Practitioners are covered under this Act as long as they act in good faith and volunteer their help; inform the person that they are a Sports First Aid Practitioner; obtain permission from the person they are helping; use reasonable skill and care according to their level of training and do not abandon the person once their offer of help has been accepted.

The Good Samaritan Act is designed to alleviate the fear of litigation from giving first aid. The relevant Government Authority recognised that people would be more willing to help if they weren't afraid of being sued, so they devised this Act to help. The Act will generally not keep you from being sued, but is a good defence, and is usually enough to prove a lawsuit frivolous, assuming that you acted within your scope of practice in good faith, and without negligence.

Scope of Practice

- Diagnose and treat injuries according to your training level
- Inform the patient that you are a Sports First Aid Practitioner
- Call for medical assistance at the earliest possible time
- Request permission before handling or treating the patient
- For an unconscious patient, ask a bystander to observe your treatment
- For a child or young adult, include the parent, guardian or coach in your treatment
- For treatment of a member of the opposite sex, treat with respect, dignity and privacy and with their permission
- Stay with the patient at all times until medical assistance arrives and brief them regarding your treatments

- Do not abandon a patient until you are relieved by medical assistance
- Document your treatment (*see* sample form in the appendix)
- Document witness names and addresses with a contact number
- Document the names and base of the medical team that took over from you at the scene
- Keep your skills up-to-date
- Never treat any injury or illness that you are not trained to diagnose or treat

Although the Good Samaritan Act is in operation in all countries, you must consult your own Government Authority regarding the situation in your own country. As a team Sports First Aid Practitioner you must also consult your insurance company regarding the provision of your service and also adhere to the Health and Safety regulations in your country regarding first aid rooms, first aid equipment and first aid provision. It is vital to protect yourself at all times, so make the calls.

Duty of Care

The duty of care that a Sports First Aid Practitioner owes to his patient is a duty to take reasonable care to avoid acts or omissions that could expose them to a reasonably foreseeable risk of injury.

The club has the same duty, but with wider responsibilities. These entail ensuring adequate supervision, safe equipment and premises, emergency policy and emergency action plan, as well as the provision of a first aid room and equipment and to comply with all Health and Safety regulations as set down by the Authority in their country.

The duty of care will arise whenever athletes are at their club or travelling to another club to participate in games or practice sessions.

A duty to take reasonable care to safeguard athletes from harm may arise before or after games or practice sessions. When dealing with children, coaches should advise parents of the exact time that supervision is available at games and practice sessions.

Away Game Activity

The club and coaches are under the same duty of care towards their athletes on an away game basis as they are at their own club.

For Children

The coach would be expected to maintain discipline sufficiently to prevent harm coming to the young athletes while on the trip and also while travelling to and from it. This may mean that additional coaches or parents will be needed to keep control, particularly if he is driving.

As a general principle, coaches have an obligation to make sure that all transport arrangements are reasonably safe and suitable to the club's requirements. Using a reputable contractor will normally ensure this.

There is a duty to take reasonable care to prevent injury through the occurrence of a reasonably foreseeable risk. In all sport there is a foreseeable risk of injury; indeed, such a risk is present in almost everything we do in our every day lives. However, the rough and tumble of physical contact is an accepted part of life, not least in growing up and developing experience and character. Clearly it would not be reasonable to prevent children from taking part in sport because there is some chance of injury.

The duty to take reasonable care is likely to be discharged by the responsible teacher ensuring that the child is not exposed to risks to which, because of some known or apparent physical illness, defect or characteristic, he is unsuited.

As part of a coach's duty of care they are obliged to attempt to assist children who are injured or sick. It is imperative that coaches remember to keep their first aid up-to-date otherwise negligence may arise because of action being taken or not being taken in these situations.

Remember

Keep your first aid up-to-date and provide young athletes and their parents with the security that a trained Sports First Aid Practitioner is standing by to assist their child if they get hurt. If your club are holding a first aid training course, invite some parents to participate in this training and assist coaches to provide a better first aid service for the young athletes.

Sports First Aid Kit

The following kit is just a recommendation of supplies you should have in your first aid kit. Various sports will require different tapes for strapping etc. so you can use this as a guideline to help you stock your own kit.

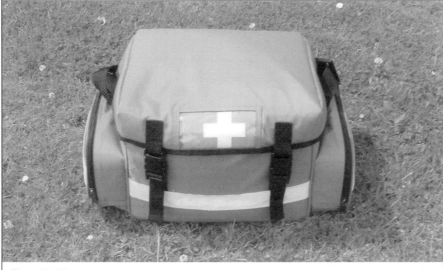

First Aid Kit.

Sports First Aid Kit Contents

Assorted Clear Waterproof Sterile Plasters	**100**
Cleaning Wipes	**100**
Wound Dressings	**12** (small, medium, large)
Protective Gloves	**20** pairs
Adhesive Dressings (7.5cm x 8cm)	**10**
Non Adherent Dressings (10cm x 10cm)	**10**
Non Adherent Dressings (5cm x 5cm)	**10**
Instant Cold Pack	**5**
Eye Wash Solution	**5** single dose bottles
Triangular Bandage–Calico	**10**
Mouth-to-mouth Resuscitation Aids	
Crépe Bandage (7.5cm x 4.5m)	**5**
Crépe Bandage (5cm x 4.5m)	**5**
Conforming Bandage (7.5cm x 4.5m)	**5**
Conforming Bandage (5cm x 4.5m)	**5**
Fabric Dressing Strip (7.5cm x 1m)	**2**
Sterile Finger Dressing	
Paramedic Shears	
Strapping Tape	**10**
Micropore Tape	**5**
Petroleum Jelly	**1** jar
Waste Bag	
Disposable Apron	
Bottle of Water	
Blanket	
Freeze Spray or Cold Gel (for acute injuries)	
Refreshing Gel (for chronic injuries)	
Blood Pressure Monitor	
SAM® Splint pack of 4	(finger, small, medium, large). Highly recommended

First Aid Room

This room should be clearly marked as a First Aid Room and should be located in an area that is accessible to people with disabilities and ambulance personnel. It should be clean, warm and properly lit as doctors or ambulance personnel may need to work on a patient. The room should have an appointed person who is responsible for the upkeep and stocking of this room and should not be locked at any time when training sessions or games are in progress. You will need to check with your Health and Safety Authority to confirm the exact requirements for your country and for the size of your club in order to comply with the regulations. Here are some of the basic requirements that are essential in a First Aid Room.

- Treatment bed
- Portable stretcher
- Hot and cold running water
- Disposable towel dispenser stocked
- Antiseptic liquid soap dispenser stocked
- Telephone
- Emergency telephone number chart
- Blankets
- Pillows
- First Aid cabinet (stocked according to Health and Safety Regulations for your club)
- Protective equipment: gloves, face masks, CPR shields and goggles
- Injury report forms and pens
- Table and chair

Emergency Telephone Number Chart

This chart should be clearly printed and framed to protect it and should be mounted beside the telephone. As a Sports First Aid Practitioner you should familiarise yourself with this chart and keep a duplicate copy in your kit bag so that you can telephone from the pitch if necessary.

Emergency Services	999 or 112
Fire Brigade	Local Base
Ambulance Control	Local Base
General Practitioner	Local Area
	On-call Service
Hospital	Casualty Unit
Neuromuscular Therapist	Local Area
Physiotherapist	Local Area
Dentist	Local Area
	On-call Service

While obtaining these numbers you should contact the professionals and discuss their referral systems, hours of practice, and emergency contact details. This will assist you in making referrals for on-going treatment for the athletes.

Pre-event Checklist

It is vital that you check the following before a game and not during an emergency when someone's life may depend on your quick response.

Things to Do

Ensure that the treatment room is clean and tidy:

- Turn on the heat
- Ensure that blankets and pillows are dry and clean
- Check the room for supplies
- Check your kit for supplies
- Check that the treatment room telephone and your mobile phone are both working
- Wear proper clothing to suit the weather
- If either a doctor or ambulance are on duty, introduce yourself and show them to the treatment room
- Meet with the game officials (referee etc.) to discuss call on protocols for the game
- Stand where you can be seen (on the sideline)

2. Introduction to First Aid

What is First Aid?

First aid is the first assistance given to a victim of a sudden accident or sudden illness.

The aims of first aid are:

- To preserve life
- To promote recovery
- To prevent the condition worsening
- To protect yourself and your patient at all times

Responsibilities of the Sports First Aid Practitioner are to:

- Respond promptly to the scene of an accident or sudden illness
- Ensure your own safety
- Protect patient(s) from further harm
- Call for appropriate help (Ambulance / Doctor / Police)
- Perform patient assessment
- Provide emergency medical care and reassurance
- Move patients only when necessary
- Take charge of the situation
- Brief EMT's (Emergency Medical Technicians) and paramedics on their arrival
- Document the care given
- Keep your knowledge and skills up-to-date

On Arrival at the Scene

- Approach carefully, ensuring no further danger to you or the patient
- Commence the primary survey
- Commence the secondary survey
- Make a diagnosis

- Give appropriate treatment
- Reassure the patient at all times
- Record all vital signs and treatments that you administered
- Call for medical assistance or arrange transport of the patient if minor

Primary Survey

A – Check the airway
B – Check the breathing and bleeding
C – Check the circulation (pulse) and the C spine
D – Disability of the patient (injury assessment)
E – Eye / ear check
F – Fractures
G – General examination

Secondary Survey

- Re-check vital signs
- Assess and diagnose injuries in priority
- Control bleeding
- Immobilize fractures
- Cover patient with a blanket
- Reassure patient
- Loosen any tight clothing (neck, chest, and waist)
- Commence a comprehensive body check
- Treat any secondary injuries
- Check vital signs again
- Arrange for medical assistance or transport to hospital

Body Check

Signs and Symptoms

- Vital signs consist of respiration, pulse, and temperature
- Signs are what you see (blood, bruising, swelling, etc.)
- Symptoms are what the patient feels (pain, tenderness, cold, etc.)

Breathing

- Normal adult resting rate is 12–20 breaths per minute
- Check rate and quality
- Look, Listen and Feel (*see* photograph 1)

Pulse

- A wave of pressure, which passes along the arteries and is created by each heart beat
- Pulse indicates speed and force of the blood in the arteries
- Three common pulse points:
    - (i) Radial (wrist)
    - (ii) Carotid (neck) (*see* photograph 2)
    - (iii) Brachial (arm)
- Take the radial pulse of a conscious patient
- Take the carotid pulse of an unconscious patient
- Normal adult resting rate is 60–80 beats per minute

Capillary refill

- The ability of the circulatory system to return blood to the capillary vessels after the blood has been squeezed out
- Most common test area is the fingertips (squeeze the fingertip for a few seconds and then release the pressure. The tip will be pale; if the refill process is working correctly then colour should return quickly to normal)

Skin condition

- Check the pallor and moisture (cold and clammy)
- Check temperature

Pupil size and reactivity (*see* photograph 3)

- Pupils of unequal size indicate an injury to the brain
- Pupils that remain constricted are often present in a person who is taking narcotics
- Pupils that remain dilated (enlarged) indicate a relaxed or unconscious state

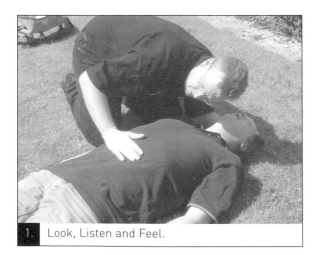
1. Look, Listen and Feel.

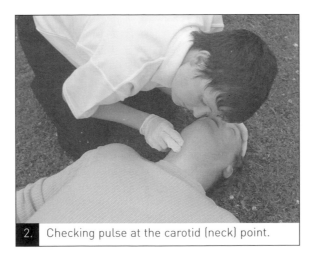
2. Checking pulse at the carotid (neck) point.

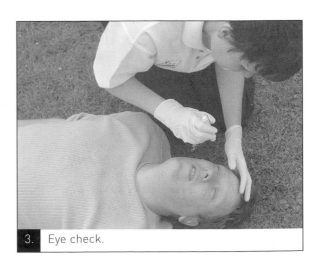
3. Eye check.

Level of consciousness

Determine using the **AVPU** scale

A – Alert
V – Responds to verbal stimuli
P – Responds to pain stimuli
U – Unconscious

Inspect for signs of injury

• Blood loss
• Deformity
• Irregularity
• Swelling

Ask the patient for symptoms

• Pain
• Dampness
• Loss of movement
• Loss of sensation

Examining the Patient from Head to Toe

Conduct a thorough hands-on examination of the:

Head
• Examine thoroughly all areas of the scalp
• Check the eye response
• Check the ears for fluid loss
• Check the nose for deformity or fluid loss
• Check the mouth for broken teeth, blood or foreign objects
• Check for any unusual odours from the breath (alcohol, sweet smell)

Neck (C spine) (*see* photograph 4)
• Gently palpate each vertebra to see whether there is pain
• Examine the neck for swelling or bleeding
• Check for the presence of an emergency medical identification neck chain

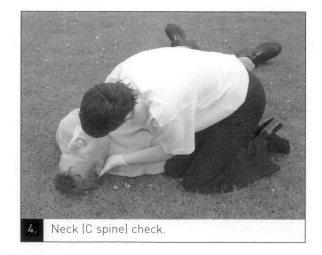

4.   Neck (C spine) check.

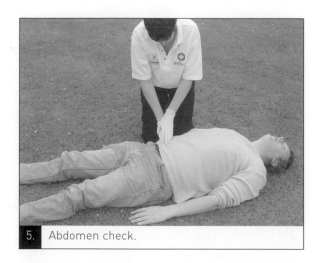

5.   Abdomen check.

Face

- Note the pallor and temperature of skin
- Note whether it is moist or dry

Chest

- Determine if the patient has difficulty breathing or coughing
- Unequal motion could be the sign of a serious condition

Abdomen (*see* photograph 5)

- Look for signs of external bleeding, penetrating injuries, or protruding parts
- Observe whether the stomach is rigid or swollen
- Divide into quarters and palpate gently; check for pain from the patient

Pelvis

- Gently press on pelvic bones
- Check for any urine that may have been passed
- Check for any stools that may have been passed
- Check for any bleeding (penal, vaginal or rectal)

Back

- Check one side of the back at a time (use the body's natural hollows)

The Extremities

- Look for bleeding and deformity
- Examine for tenderness
- Ask the patient to move the extremity
- Check for sensation
- Assess the circulatory status (distal pulse–capillary refill)

The Patient's Medical History

Using the **SAMPLE** scale, shown below, it is important to gather as much information as possible. This will assist doctors in their treatment later.

S – Signs / symptoms
A – Allergies
M – Medications
P – Past medical history
L – Last oral intake
E – Events leading to or associated with the illness or injury

Shock

This is a state in which the circulatory system fails to supply enough blood to peripheral tissues of the body to meet basic requirements. Most medical emergencies include a victim suffering from shock. Knowing how to treat and diagnose a person in shock is a very important first aid tool. Shock can be as minor as feeling faint or as severe as depressing the major body organs like the heart and lungs from working normally. Therefore, severe shock can lead to death if not treated correctly.

Signs and Symptoms of Shock

- Confusion, restlessness, anxiety
- Pale skin with a cold clammy sweat
- Rapid, weak pulse
- Rapid shallow breathing
- Thirst, nausea, vomiting
- General weakness, feel like fainting

Treatment of Shock

• Position the patient correctly (if unconscious, use recovery position)

• Place a blanket over the patient

• Loosen any tight clothing (neck, chest and waist)

• Maintain the patient's vitals

• Control bleeding

• Cover the patient with a blanket

• Do not give the patient anything to eat or drink

• Arrange transport to hospital

3. The Circulatory System, Wounds and Bleeding

The Circulatory System

The circulatory system includes the heart, the blood, the arteries, the veins and the capillaries. The blood is the transport system by which oxygen and nutrients travel through the body, reach the body's cells and waste materials are carried away. In addition, blood carries substances called hormones, which control body processes, and antibodies to fight invading germs. The heart, a muscular organ, positioned behind the ribcage and between the lungs, is the pump that keeps this transport system moving.

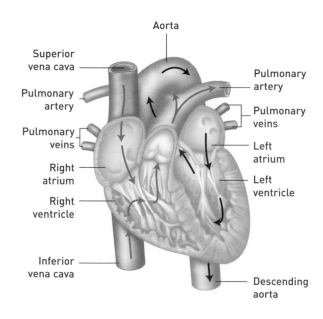

Figure 3.1: The heart.

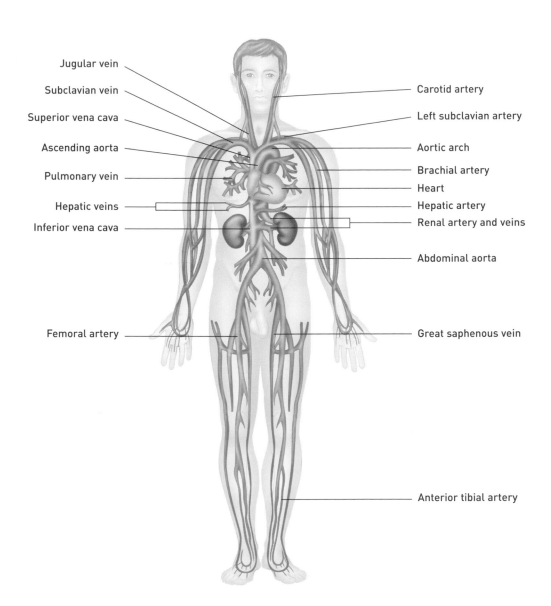

Figure 3.2: The cardiovascular system.

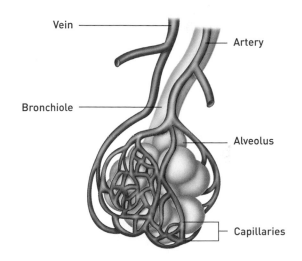

Figure 3.3: Arteries, veins, and capillaries.

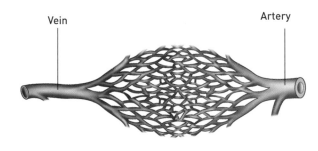

Figure 3.4: A capillary.

The Blood Vessels

Blood vessels are hollow tubes forming the pipework of the circulatory system. The walls have an outer layer of connective tissue, a middle layer of smooth muscle, and an inner layer of epidermal tissue.

Arteries carry rich oxygenated blood away from the heart and deliver oxygen to all tissues in the body. Arteries are thick walled vessels.

Veins carry de-oxygenated blood to the heart. Veins are thin walled vessels and have a one-way valve to ensure that the flow of blood is towards the heart.

Capillaries allow oxygen to be supplied to tissues and muscles and carbon dioxide to be collected. Capillaries are thin walled thread-like vessels.

The Blood

An average person has about 4–5 litres of blood that consists of 55% liquid plasma and 45% blood cells. As described above, blood is responsible for carrying oxygen, carbon dioxide, water, glucose, waste matter, and heat throughout the body. Blood may also carry organisms that cause diseases such as Hepatitis B Virus (HBV) and Human Immuno-deficiency Virus (HIV), which are transmitted from an infected person's blood, semen and / or vaginal fluids. These organisms may also enter through cuts or breaks in your skin or through the lining of your mouth, nose, and eyes.

Bleeding

There are three types of bleeding:

1. Arterial (severe) – Blood that comes from an artery. It is bright red in colour (because it is full of oxygen) and will spurt from a wound.
2. Venous (moderate) – Blood that comes from a vein. It is dark red in colour (because it is full of carbon dioxide) and will flow from a wound.
3. Capillary (minor) – Blood that comes from a capillary. It is a brick red colour (because it has both oxygen and carbon dioxide) and will ooze from a wound.

Precautions

As we saw above, any infection may enter our bodies through cuts, breaks in the skin, through the mouth and nose or by being splashed in the eyes. The following gear / precautions should be worn / taken:

• Protective gloves

• Goggles

• Face mask

• CPR shield

• Cover the victim's open wounds with dressings, extra gauze or waterproof material

• Use a mouth-to-mouth barrier device when you do rescue breathing. The victim could have blood in the mouth or may vomit

• Wash your hands with soap and water immediately

• In any incident where you are exposed to a victim's blood or other body fluids, seek medical advise a.s.a.p.

Wounds

A wound is the tearing of the skin, tissues or muscles of the body. Once this occurs the wound allows blood to flow out and germs to enter the body. The two main objectives with any wounds should be:

1. Blood loss control – Controlling bleeding by direct or indirect pressure, the application of a sterile dressing and securing a bandage in place
2. Infection control – It is vital to firstly, protect yourself. Wearing your protective equipment (gloves, goggles, face mask), sterilise the area of injury and only use sterile dressings and bandages. Although you may feel silly wearing all this equipment, you should never risk becoming infected.

A closed wound will be caused by impact to the body. It can range from a minor bruise or sprain, to a skull fracture with brain damage or a spinal cord injury with paralysis.

An open wound is caused when the skin and under-lying tissue is torn away. Foreign matter such as bacteria, dirt, and clothing fragments may enter the body and cause infection. Other factors affecting severity include depth, surface area and structures that become damaged. Infection control is vital in the case of any wound to the body.

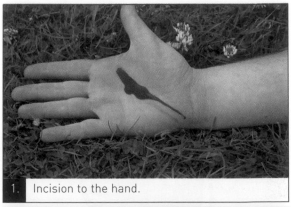
1. Incision to the hand.

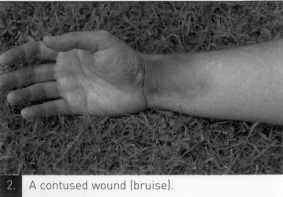
2. A contused wound (bruise).

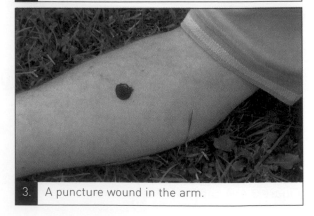
3. A puncture wound in the arm.

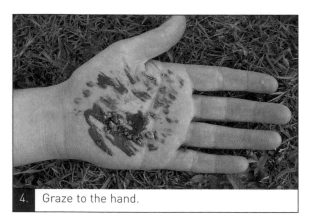

4. Graze to the hand.

Wound Types

- Incised   A clean cut caused by a sharp edged object (knife) (*see* photograph 1)
- Contused   A closed wound (bruise) caused by a blow from a blunt object (hammer) (*see* photograph 2)
- Laceration   A rough tearing of the skin and soft tissue caused by a jagged edged object (bull-wire)
- Punctured   A wound caused by a sharp pointed object (nail) (*see* photograph 3)
- Graze   A scrapping of the dermis caused by friction (*see* photograph 4)
- Shot   A small entry and large exit wound caused by a bullet entering the body

External Bleeding

External bleeding is caused by a tearing of the skin covering, tissues or muscles and allows blood to flow out of the body.

Signs and Symptoms of External Bleeding

- History of an accident
- Blood visible at the site of the wound (bright red, spurting – arterial);

(dark red, flows – venous)
- Patient's face will be pale
- Patient will have cold, clammy skin
- Pulse will be rapid and weak
- Patient will feel faint and dizzy
- Patient will feel nauseous and may vomit
- Patient will be thirsty
- Patient may become unconscious
- Shock

Treatment of External Bleeding

- Put on your protective gear (gloves, face mask, and goggles)
- Apply direct pressure on the wound (if no foreign body is imbedded)
- Apply a sterile dressing
- Secure dressing with a bandage (roller or triangular)
- Elevate the injured limb
- If bleeding persists, place another dressing and bandage over the first one. Do not remove the original dressing or bandage
- Cover the patient with a blanket for shock
- Reassure the patient at all times
- Monitor vital signs
- If the patient becomes unconscious, place them in the recovery position
- Call for medical assistance or arrange transport to hospital if minor

Internal Bleeding

Bleeding which occurs within the body.

Signs and Symptoms of Internal Bleeding

- History of an accident
- Patient may be in pain
- Patient may have pattern of bruising
- Patient's face will be pale

- Patient will have cold, clammy skin
- Pulse will be rapid and weak
- Breathing will be rapid and may be laboured
- Patient will feel anxious and restless
- Patient will feel nauseous and may vomit
- Patient's vital signs and conscious level may deteriorate
- Patient may become unconscious
- Shock
- Blood may become visible:
    (i) Coughing – injury to lungs
    (ii) Vomiting – injury to stomach or abdomen
    (iii) Urine – injury to kidney or bladder
    (iv) Back passage – injury to bowel
    (v) Ears – injury to brain (straw coloured fluid may be also present CSF)

Treatment of Internal Bleeding

- Put on your protective gear (gloves, face mask, and goggles)
- Lie the patient down in a comfortable position
- Cover with a blanket
- Loosen all tight clothing (neck, chest, and waist)
- Raise the patient's legs
- Cover the patient with a blanket for shock
- Reassure the patient at all times
- Monitor vital signs
- If the patient becomes unconscious, place them in the recovery position
- Call for medical assistance

Control Methods

1. Direct pressure – Pressure applied directly over the wound to stop blood flow
2. Indirect pressure – Pressure applied to the artery superior to a wound site to stop blood flow (e.g. wound to lower arms – pressure to brachial artery)

Treatment and Bandaging of Wounds and Bleeding

Wound with Capillary Bleeding

- Irrigate the wound with sterile water
- Place a sterile dressing over the wound site
- Place cotton wool or gauze padding on the dressing
- Apply a compression roller bandage
- Elevate the limb (if no under-lying fractures are present)
- Refer to hospital

Wound with Venous or Arterial Bleeding

- Apply a sterile dressing to the wound
- Apply direct pressure with your hand over the dressing
- Raise the limb (if no under-lying fractures are present)
- Apply a compression roller bandage
- Call for medical assistance

4. Basic Life Support

Respiration is achieved through the mouth, nose, trachea, lungs, and diaphragm. Oxygen enters the respiratory system through the mouth and the nose. The oxygen then passes through the larynx (where speech sounds are produced) and the trachea, which is a tube that enters the chest cavity.

In the chest cavity, the trachea splits into two smaller tubes called the *bronchi*. Each bronchus then divides again forming the bronchial tubes. The bronchial tubes lead directly into the lungs where they divide into many smaller tubes, which connect to tiny sacs, called *alveoli*. The average adult's lungs contain about 600 million of these spongy, air-filled sacs that are surrounded by capillaries. The inhaled oxygen passes into the alveoli and then diffuses through the capillaries into the arterial blood. Meanwhile, the waste-rich blood from the veins releases its carbon dioxide into the alveoli. The carbon dioxide follows the same path out of the lungs when you exhale.

The *diaphragm* is a sheet of muscle that lies across the bottom of the chest cavity. The diaphragm's job is to help pump the carbon dioxide out of the lungs and pull the oxygen into the lungs. As the diaphragm contracts and relaxes, breathing takes place. When the diaphragm contracts, oxygen is pulled into the lungs. When the diaphragm relaxes, carbon dioxide is pumped out of the lungs. If the body is prevented from completing this action, then as a Sports First Aid Practitioner you must commence Basic Life Support (BLS) to facilitate this process and maintain oxygen to the brain and vital organs.

Heart attacks (or myocardial infarctions) have become a common cause of sudden death in sporting events in recent years. A key task for a Sports First Aid Practitioner is to provide early access to Basic Life Support for the victim of a heart attack whilst waiting for ambulance personnel to arrive.

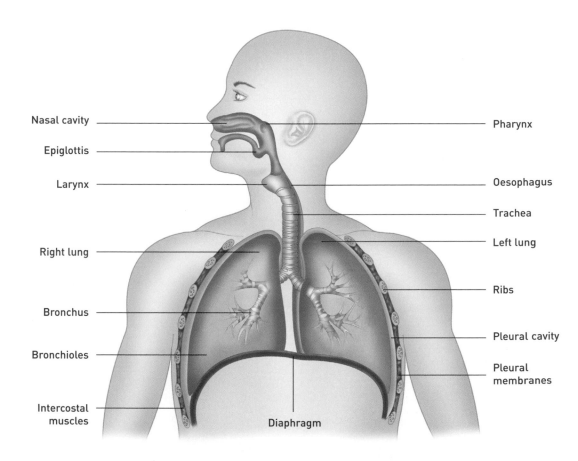

Figure 4.1: The respiratory system.

Inhalation

Exhalation

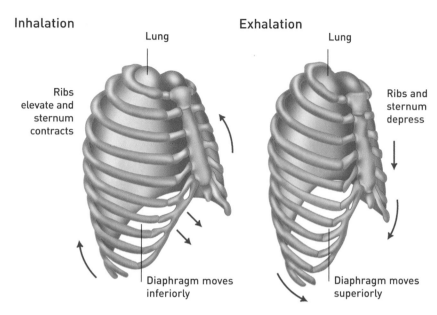

Figure 4.2: The mechanics of respiration.

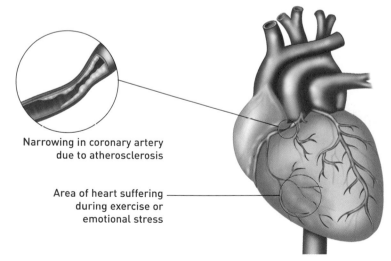

Narrowing in coronary artery
due to atherosclerosis

Area of heart suffering
during exercise or
emotional stress

Figure 4.3: Angina.

The Heart

The heart is an involuntary muscular pump, which pumps blood around the body (see figure 3.1). There are some heart conditions of which you must be aware.

Angina

Angina leads to severe chest pain as there is insufficient blood supply getting to the heart muscles. The condition is normally brought on by exercise, physical or emotional stress, but will improve with rest.

Signs and Symptoms of Angina

- Gripping chest pain may extend to the neck, shoulder and arm
- Tingling sensation in the hand
- Air hunger (gasping for air)
- Face may be ashen in pallor
- Lips may be cyanosed (blue)
- Pain will decrease with rest and medication
- An attack may last between 3–8 minutes
- Patient may become unconscious
- Shock

Treatment of Angina

- Place the patient in a comfortable lying position
- Cover the patient with a blanket
- Loosen tight clothing (neck, chest and waist)
- Encourage the patient to take their medication (spray, tablet)
- Reassure the patient
- Be prepared to give BLS
- Call for a cardiac ambulance
- Monitor and record vital signs

Heart Attack

This condition is caused when a coronary artery becomes blocked causing an insufficient blood supply to the heart, which leads to damage to the heart muscles. This blockage may be due to a clot in the artery (coronary thrombosis) or a fatty substance build up in the artery (atherosclerosis).

Signs and Symptoms of a Heart Attack

- Constant crushing chest pain
- Air hunger (gasping for air)
- Superior abdomen discomfort (like severe indigestion)
- Patient may feel an impending sense of doom
- Face may be ashen in pallor
- Lips may be cyanosed (blue)
- Pulse will become rapid, and weaker
- Patient may feel giddy or faint
- Patient may become unconscious
- Breathing and circulation may stop
- Shock

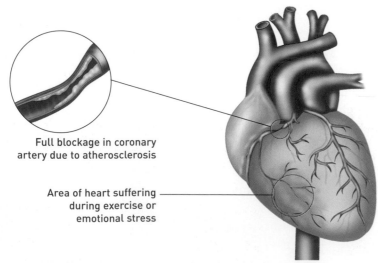

Full blockage in coronary artery due to atherosclerosis

Area of heart suffering during exercise or emotional stress

Figure 4.4: Heart attack.

Treatment of a Heart Attack

- Place the patient in a half sitting position (use blankets, etc. to prop the patient up)
- Loosen tight clothing (neck, chest and waist)
- Cover the patient with a blanket
- Call for a cardiac ambulance
- Be prepared to give BLS
- Monitor and record vital signs

Cardiac Arrest

This condition occurs when the heart stops beating completely and may be caused by drowning, poisoning, or a heart attack.

Signs and Symptoms of a Cardiac Arrest

- Patient will be unconscious
- Patient will be unresponsive
- Breathing will be absent
- Pulse will be absent
- Shock

Treatment of a Cardiac Arrest

- Call for a cardiac ambulance
- Commence CPR (Cardiopulmonary Resuscitation)

Adult CPR

1. Check scene safety
2. Shake and shout (hello, can you hear me) (no response)
3. Call for a cardiac ambulance
4. Open the airway (head tilt – chin lift) (*see* photograph 1)
5. Check for breathing (look, listen and feel); 10 seconds (no response)
6. Apply CPR shield (*see* photograph 2)

7. Give two rescue breaths (*see* photograph 3)

8. Check pulse (carotid); 10 seconds (no response) (*see* photograph 4)

9. Locate your hand position (locate the inferior point of sternum, measure two fingers above and place the heel of your hand on site)

10. Commence chest compressions (15 – at a rate of 1 and 2 and 3 etc. at a depth of 1–1.5"; 4cm to 5cm) (*see* photograph 5)

11. Repeat steps 6–9

12. Continue for 4 cycles (finish on 2 rescue breaths)

13. Check pulse (carotid)

14. Resume chest compressions (check vital signs after 3 minutes)

15. If the patient resumes breathing and the pulse returns, place in the recovery position (*see* page 40)

16. Maintain an open airway (in case of vomiting, swallowing of the tongue)

17. Monitor and record vital signs

18. Loosen tight clothing (neck, chest and waist)

19. Cover the patient with a blanket

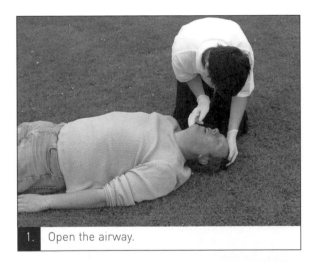
1. Open the airway.

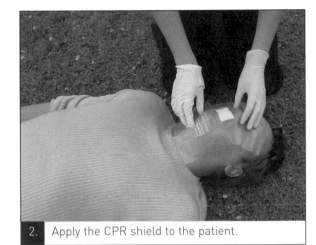
2. Apply the CPR shield to the patient.

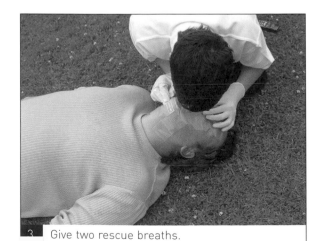
3. Give two rescue breaths.

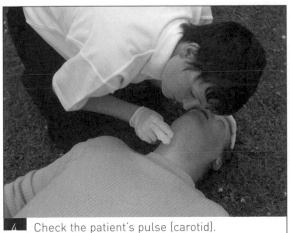
4. Check the patient's pulse (carotid).

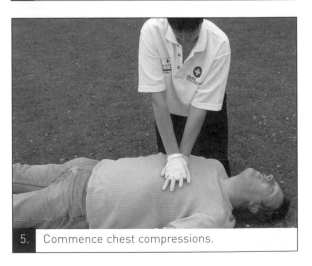
5. Commence chest compressions.

Child CPR (1–8 years)

1. Check scene safety
2. Shake and shout (hello, can you hear me) (no response) (see photograph 1)
3. Open the airway (head tilt – chin lift) (see photograph 2)
4. Check for breathing (look, listen and feel); 10 seconds (no response) (see photograph 3)
5. Apply CPR shield (see photograph 4)
6. Give two rescue breaths (see photograph 5)
7. Check pulse (carotid); 10 seconds (no response) (see photograph 6)

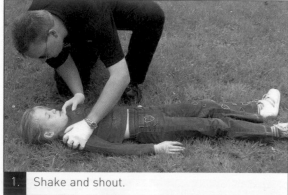

1. Shake and shout.

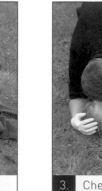

2. Open the airway.

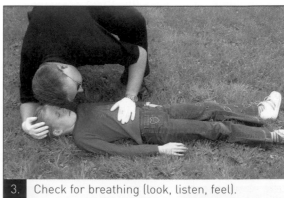

3. Check for breathing (look, listen, feel).

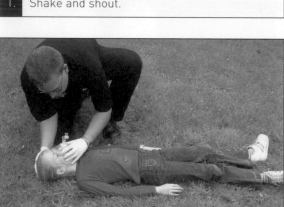

4. Apply the CPR shield to the patient.

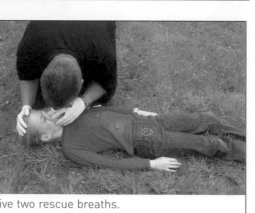

5. Give two rescue breaths.

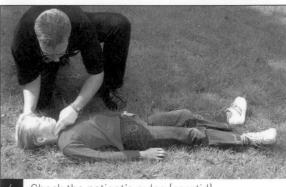

6. Check the patient's pulse (carotid).

8. Locate your hand position (locate the inferior point of sternum, measure two fingers above and place heel of your hand on site) (one hand at a depth of 1-1.5"; 2.5cm–4cm) (*see* photograph 7)

9. Commence chest compressions (5 – at a rate of 1, 2, 3 etc.) (*see* photograph 8)

10. Repeat sleps 5–8 twenty times

11. Call for a cardiac ambulance

12. Check pulse (carotid)

13. Resume chest compressions (check vital signs after 3 minutes)

14. If the patient resumes breathing and the pulse returns, place in the recovery position (*see* page 40)

15. Maintain an open airway (in case of vomiting, swallowing of the tongue) (*see* photograph 9)

16. Monitor and record vital signs

17. Loosen tight clothing (neck, chest and waist)

18. Cover the patient with a blanket

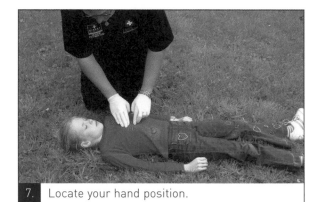

7. Locate your hand position.

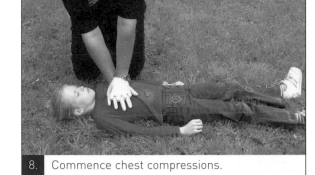

8. Commence chest compressions.

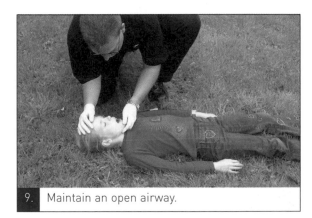

9. Maintain an open airway.

Adult Foreign Body Airway Obstruction (FBAO) (Conscious)

1. Check scene safety
2. Are you choking? Can you speak?
   (see photograph 1)
3. Can you cough? (If yes, encourage to do so)

If object does not dislodge with coughing:

4. Go behind the patient
5. Make a fist and place it between the naval and the inferior point of sternum
6. Place second hand on fist
7. Give 5 abdominal thrusts (bring hands inwards and upwards) (see photograph 2)
8. Continue until object is dislodged
9. If patient becomes unconscious, commence steps for FBAO unconscious patient from step 3 below (see photographs 3 & 4)

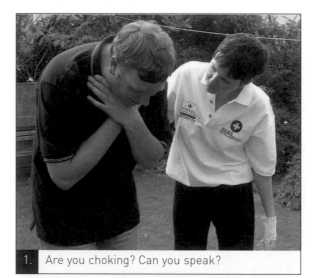

1. Are you choking? Can you speak?

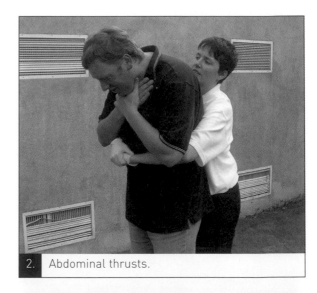

2. Abdominal thrusts.

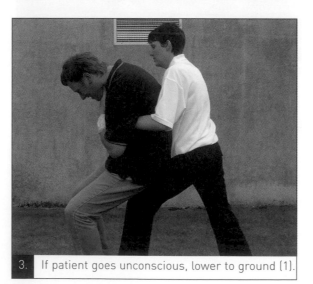

3. If patient goes unconscious, lower to ground (1).

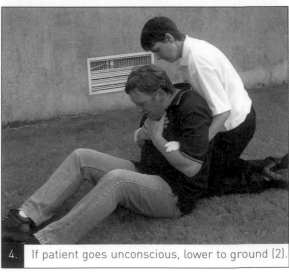

4. If patient goes unconscious, lower to ground (2).

Adult Foreign Body Airway Obstruction (Unconscious)

1. Check scene safety
2. Shake and shout (hello, can you hear me) (no response)
3. Call for a cardiac ambulance (*see* photograph 1)
4. Open the airway (head tilt – chin lift) (*see* photograph 2)
5. Check for breathing (look, listen and feel); 10 seconds (no response)
6. Apply CPR shield (*see* photograph 3)
7. Give rescue breaths (if unsuccessful, reposition the head and try again) (*see* photograph 4)
8. If unsuccessful, straddle the patient and give 5 abdominal thrusts (*see* photograph 5)
9. Open the airway (tongue, jaw lift) (*see* photograph 6)
10. Carry out a blind finger sweep
11. Repeat steps 6–9 until object is dislodged

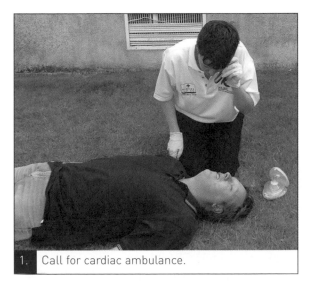

1. Call for cardiac ambulance.

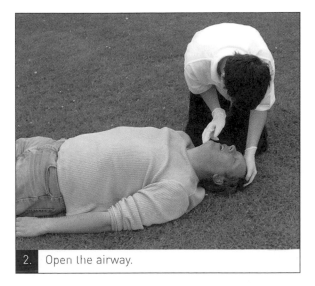

2. Open the airway.

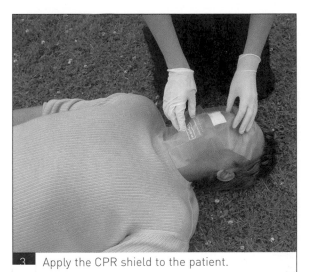

3. Apply the CPR shield to the patient.

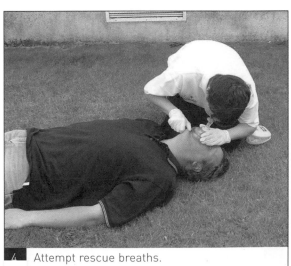

4. Attempt rescue breaths.

Adult Foreign Body Airway Obstruction (Unconscious) *(continued)*

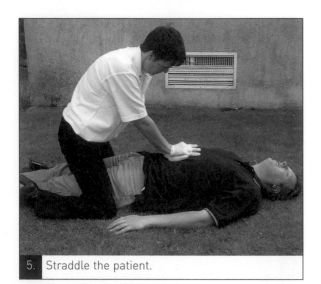

5. Straddle the patient.

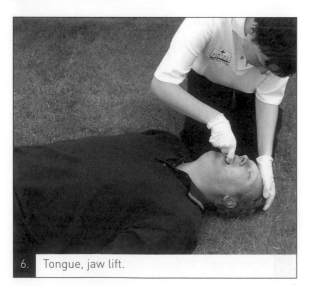

6. Tongue, jaw lift.

Child Foreign Body Airway Obstruction (Conscious)

1. Check scene safety
2. Are you choking? Can you speak?
   (*see* photograph 1)
3. Can you cough? (if yes, encourage to do so)

If object does not dislodge with coughing:

4. Go behind the patient
5. Make a fist and place it between the naval and the inferior point of sternum
6. Give 5 abdominal thrusts (bring hands inwards and upwards) (*see* photograph 2)
7. Continue until object is dislodged
8. If patient becomes unconscious, commence steps for child FBAO unconscious patient from step 3 below (*see* photograph 3)

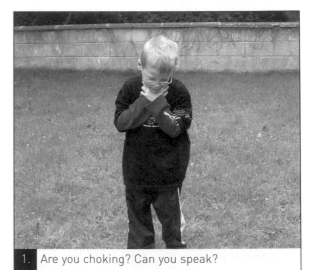

1. Are you choking? Can you speak?

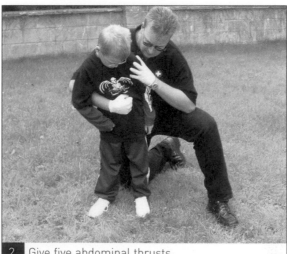

2. Give five abdominal thrusts.

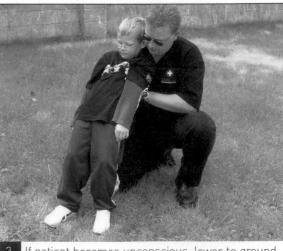

3. If patient becomes unconscious, lower to ground.

Child Foreign Body Airway Obstruction (Unconscious)

1. Check scene safety
2. Shake and shout (hello can you hear me) (no response) (*see* photograph 1)
3. Call for help – call for a cardiac ambulance (*see* photograph 2)
4. Open the airway (head tilt – chin lift)
5. Check for breathing (look, listen and feel); 10 seconds (no response)
6. Apply CPR shield
7. Give rescue breaths (if unsuccessful, reposition the head and try again) (*see* photograph 3)
8. If unsuccessful, straddle the patient and give 5 one handed abdominal thrusts (*see* photograph 4)
9. Open the airway (tongue, jaw lift, check mouth for obstruction) (*see* photograph 5, overleaf)
10. Repeat steps 6–9 until object is dislodged

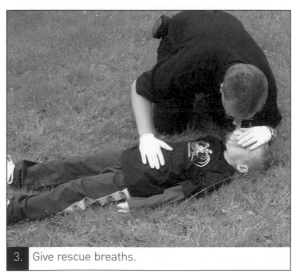

1. Shake and shout.

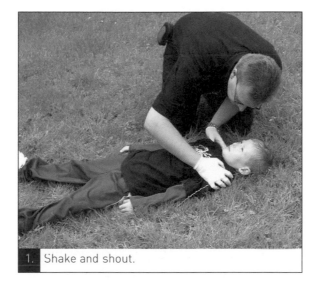

2. Call for a cardiac ambulance.

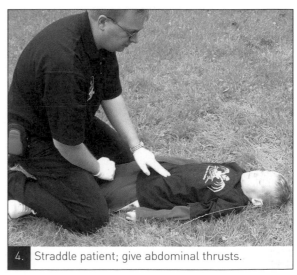

3. Give rescue breaths.

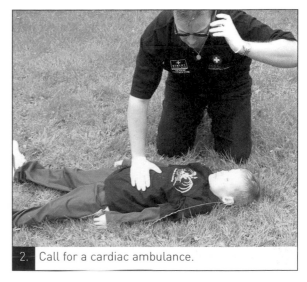

4. Straddle patient; give abdominal thrusts.

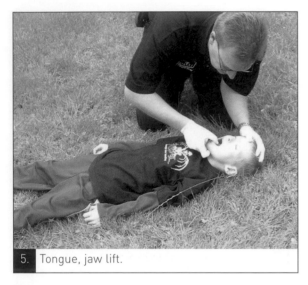

5. Tongue, jaw lift.

The Recovery Position

The recovery position may need to be used in many conditions that require first aid such as unconsciousness.

By placing the patient into this position you will:

• Maintain an open airway
• Minimise the risk of the patient being injured further
• Allow drainage from the mouth and nose

It should not be used when a person:

• Is not breathing
• Has a head, neck, or spinal injury
• Has a serious injury

The recovery position:

• Allows the victim to breathe more easily
• Maintains an open airway. It allows fluids such as vomit and blood to drain so that the victim doesn't choke on them
• Promotes good circulation throughout the body
• Supports the body in a safe position and minimises the patient injuring themselves further

To Put a Person in the Recovery Position

1. Kneel at the patient's side
2. Turn the patient's face toward you. Tilt the head back to open the airway (*see* photograph 1)
3. Check the mouth if the patient is unconscious and remove false teeth or any foreign matter
4. Place the patient's arm nearest you, with palm up into a right angle (the HOW position) (*see* photograph 2)
5. Place the patient's other arm across the chest with the fingertips resting on the shoulder, palm down (*see* photograph 3)
6. Bend the leg furthest away from you, and tuck the foot under the knee (*see* photograph 4)
7. Support the patient's head with one hand and grasp his knee furthest from you (*see* photograph 5)
8. Roll the patient towards you
9. Rest the patient against your knees
10. Bend the patient's upper arm and leg until each forms a right angle to the body. This position helps to support the patient
11. Don't let the patient roll onto his face (*see* photograph 6)
12. Make sure the head is tilted back to keep the airway open
13. Treat the patient for shock

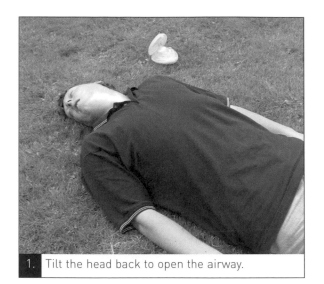

1. Tilt the head back to open the airway.

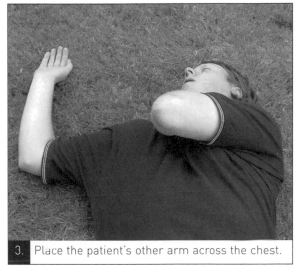

2. Place the patient's arm into the HOW position.

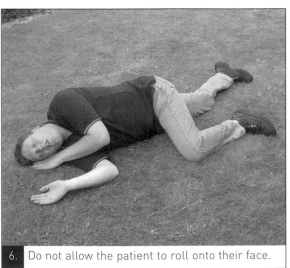

3. Place the patient's other arm across the chest.

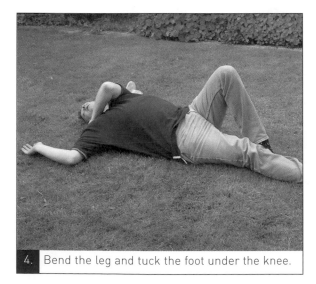

4. Bend the leg and tuck the foot under the knee.

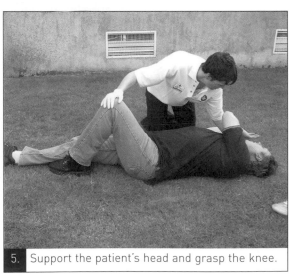

5. Support the patient's head and grasp the knee.

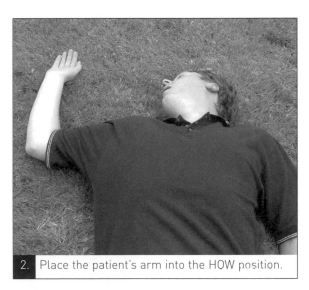

6. Do not allow the patient to roll onto their face.

Maintaining an Open Airway (*see* photograph 1)

An unconscious casualty has no control over his muscles, including the muscles that control the tongue. The relaxed tongue will fall backwards across the airway, and cause an obstruction and cut off the air supply. If a breathing unconscious casualty remains on his back, the risk of airway obstruction is increased. Care of the airway in an unconscious casualty takes precedence over any other injury or illness, including spinal injuries.

In most situations the airway can be managed with the use of backward head tilt and chin lift. In the event that a foreign body obstructs the airway, then the airway should be cleared using a finger sweep with the casualty lying on their side to avoid accidental inhalation of obstructions.

• Roll the casualty onto the (uninjured) side
• Place your hand on the forehead and gently tilt the head back (in case of spinal injury, perform a jaw thrust)
• Support and lift the chin to open the airway
• Lift the jaw forward to open the mouth
• Remove any visible obstruction from the victim's mouth
• Remove mouth shields
• Remove dislodged or loose dentures
• Leave well fitting dentures in place to maintain shape of the mouth

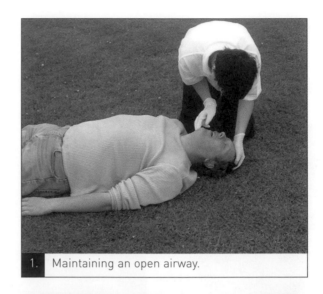

1. Maintaining an open airway.

Jaw Thrust (*see* photograph 2)

In some instances involving injuries or illness, the casualty's airway may be difficult to open. An alternative method of airway maintenance is the jaw thrust.

• Apply pressure with the fingers behind the angle of the lower jaw (inferior to ear lobe)
• Thrust the jaw gently forward and up, opening the airway

It is **vital** when performing any of these procedures that you protect yourself by wearing protective gloves and using face shields.

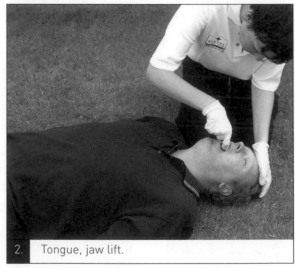

2. Tongue, jaw lift.

CPREzy – "Making CPR Easy"

Basic life support training (chest compressions and ventilations) has the same issues as any other area of training that is not used, or is used after long periods of time – primarily that people forget what to do and even when they do remember they can't apply the knowledge. Indeed the Resuscitation Council UK (RCUK) have stated that after 6 months, typically 90% of CPR training has been forgotten. Consequently, a large element of guesswork then comes into play.

CPR has its own issues in terms of good performance.

- Knowing, remembering and being able to apply and maintain the correct compression rate
- Knowing and being able to apply the correct pressure
- Too little – ineffective
- Too much – broken ribs, wasted energy etc.
- Fatigue
- CPR performance can decline as much as 80% in the first minute due to rescuer fatigue
- Skill loss

- Research confirms skill loss starting from 2 weeks
- Skill retention may be as low as 10% after 6 months (RCUK)
- Lack of confidence
- Results in fear and hesitation
- Potential health issues in providing mouth-to-mouth resuscitation
- Incorrect hand positioning
- Can result in punctured lungs
- Ineffective chest compressions

What does this all mean?

It means that although you can be sure your people have been trained, you can't be sure that they are competent. With CPREzy available, you can be sure that your First Aiders are competent in delivery of chest compressions and consequently maximise the chances of survival until the defibrillator is available.

CPREzy consists of a pad to ensure delivery of consistently effective chest compressions during cardiac arrest and training, and a mask designed to overcome the lack of confidence in delivering ventilations. It is designed to be totally complementary to existing guidelines and training (i.e. ILCOR / AHA / ERC / RCUK).

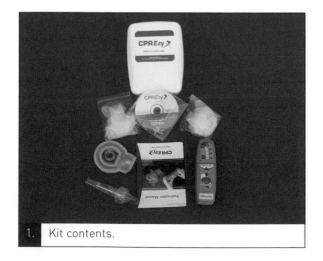

1. Kit contents.

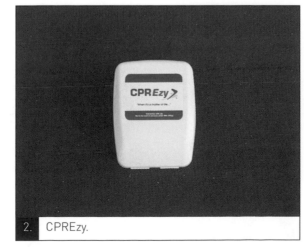

2. CPREzy.

CPREzy – Pad

• Indicates the correct force and frequency
• Visual and audible flashing metronome ensures correct rate
• LED's indicate correct pressure for correct and consistent chest compression, for different size patients
• Potentially reduces the risk of chest injury
• Assists with full release of force between compressions
• Reduces rescuer fatigue due to effectiveness of delivery
• Adds value to a training course
• Gives the rescuer confidence to perform by taking the guesswork out of chest compressions

CPREzy – Mask

• Rescuer is approximately 3ins (7.5cm) away from the face of the victim, thereby overcoming most of the reservations linked with mouth-to-mouth resuscitation
• One-way valve prevents blow-back of fluids
• Unique patient tube delivers air directly into the mouth
• Automatically blocks the victim's nose (all nose types)
• Overcomes lack of confidence to perform ventilations

Often chest compressions are not carried out, due to fear of doing mouth-to-mouth resuscitation. If this fear is overcome, it is more likely that chest compressions will also be attempted.

In the absence of a defibrillator, effective CPR is paramount to the victim's chances of survival. If CPR is not administered correctly, survival rates are considerably reduced. In summary:

• There are a great many heart attacks each year
• 90% of first aider's CPR skills are lost within 6 months
• There are problems with normal CPR performance, particularly in the application of correct compression rates and pressures
• CPREzy complements existing training and resuscitation guidelines
• Many first aiders do not have the confidence to start CPR
• CPREzy assists trained people to perform CPR correctly and raises the standard of first aid training and practice
• CPREzy should be used in conjunction with all AEDs to work towards optimal resuscitation
• Training on CPREzy is simple and available throughout the UK and Ireland by Direct First Aid UK

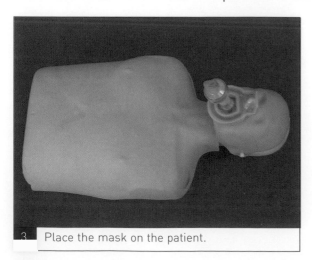

3   Place the mask on the patient.

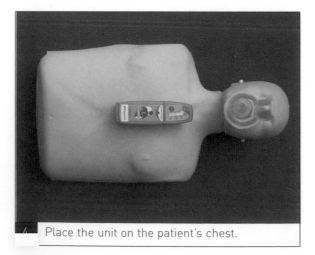

4   Place the unit on the patient's chest.

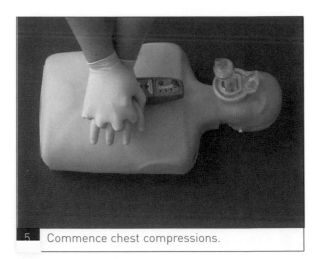

5   Commence chest compressions.

• There is no other product available in the world like CPREzy
• CPREzy increases the chances of saving a life by ensuring competency
  in delivery of chest compressions

Instructions for Use

The CPREzy is simple to use and requires very little extra training. However, each kit comes with full instructions both in a manual and on a CD-Rom. More information is available on the website www.healthaffairs.co.uk (*see* Useful Addresses).

5. Fractures and the Skeleton

The skeleton is made up of 206 bones and is responsible for:

- Providing support for the body and muscular system
- Protecting the vital organs of the body
- Providing movement in conjunction with the muscular system
- Providing shape
- Producing red blood cells through bone marrow

Axial Skeleton: Skull, Vertebrae, and Bony Thorax

Skull: consists of cranial bones and facial bones.

Cranial bones: eight large flat bones: comprising two pairs, plus four single bones.
These surround the brain and consist of: **frontal** (forms forehead); **parietal** (pair of bones); **temporal** (pair of bones); **occipital** (posterior bone of the cranium); **sphenoid** (spans the width of the skull); **ethmoid** (two lateral masses, one on each side of the nasal cavity).

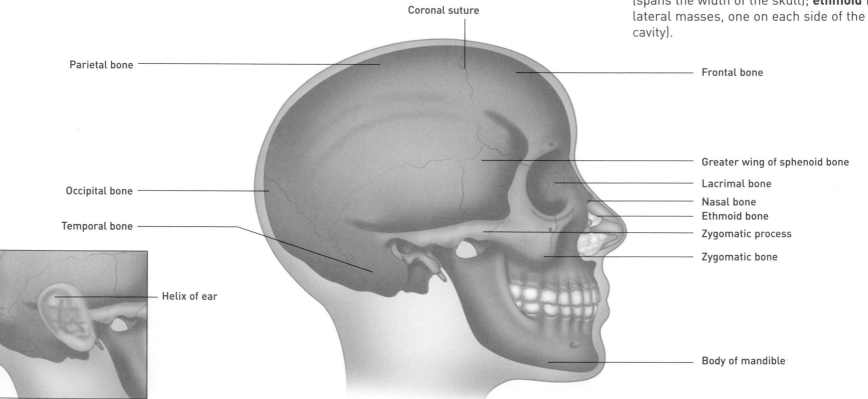

Coronal suture

Parietal bone

Occipital bone

Temporal bone

Helix of ear

Frontal bone

Greater wing of sphenoid bone

Lacrimal bone

Nasal bone

Ethmoid bone

Zygomatic process

Zygomatic bone

Body of mandible

Figure 5.1: The cranial bones.

Facial bones: make up remainder of face, comprising mandible, maxilla, palatine, zygomatic, lacrimal, nasal (also vomer and inferior nasal conchae).

a.

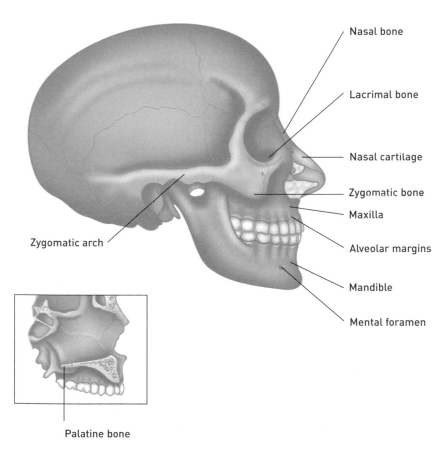

b.

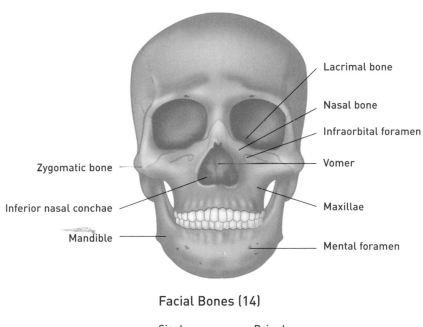

Facial Bones (14)

<u>Single</u>	<u>Paired</u>
Mandible	Maxillae
Vomer	Zygomatic
	Nasal
	Lacrimal
	Palatine
	Inferior nasal conchae

Figures 5.2a & b: The facial bones.

Vertebrae: cervical, thoracic, lumbar, sacrum, coccyx.

Bony thorax: ribs, sternum.

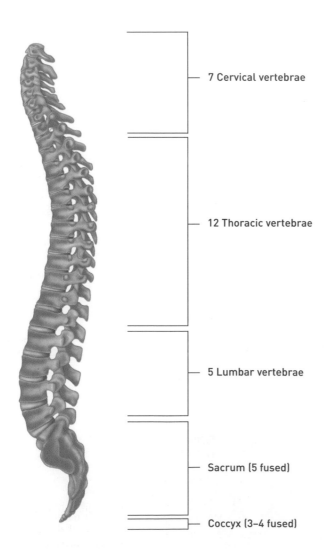

7 Cervical vertebrae

12 Thoracic vertebrae

5 Lumbar vertebrae

Sacrum (5 fused)

Coccyx (3–4 fused)

Figure 5.3: The vertebral column (spine, lateral view).

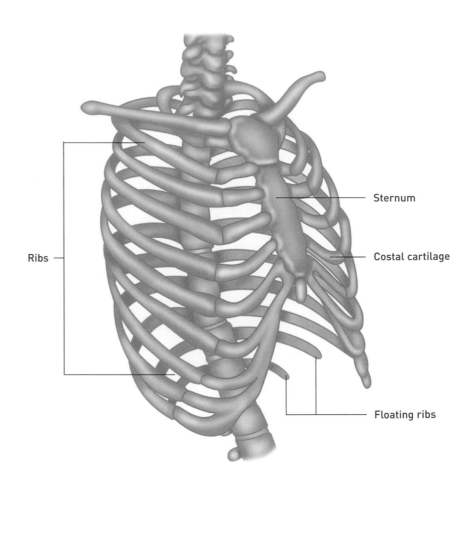

Ribs

Sternum

Costal cartilage

Floating ribs

Figure 5.4: The bony thorax.

Appendicular Skeleton: Pectoral Girdle, Arms, Pelvic Girdle, Legs

Pectoral girdle: attaches arm to axial skeleton (scapula, clavicle).

Arm bones: humerus, radius, ulna, carpals, metacarpals, and phalanges (distal, middle, and proximal).

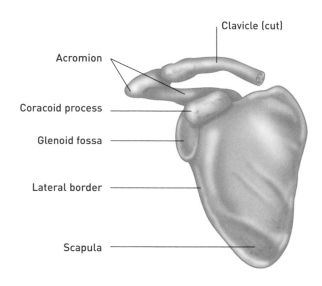

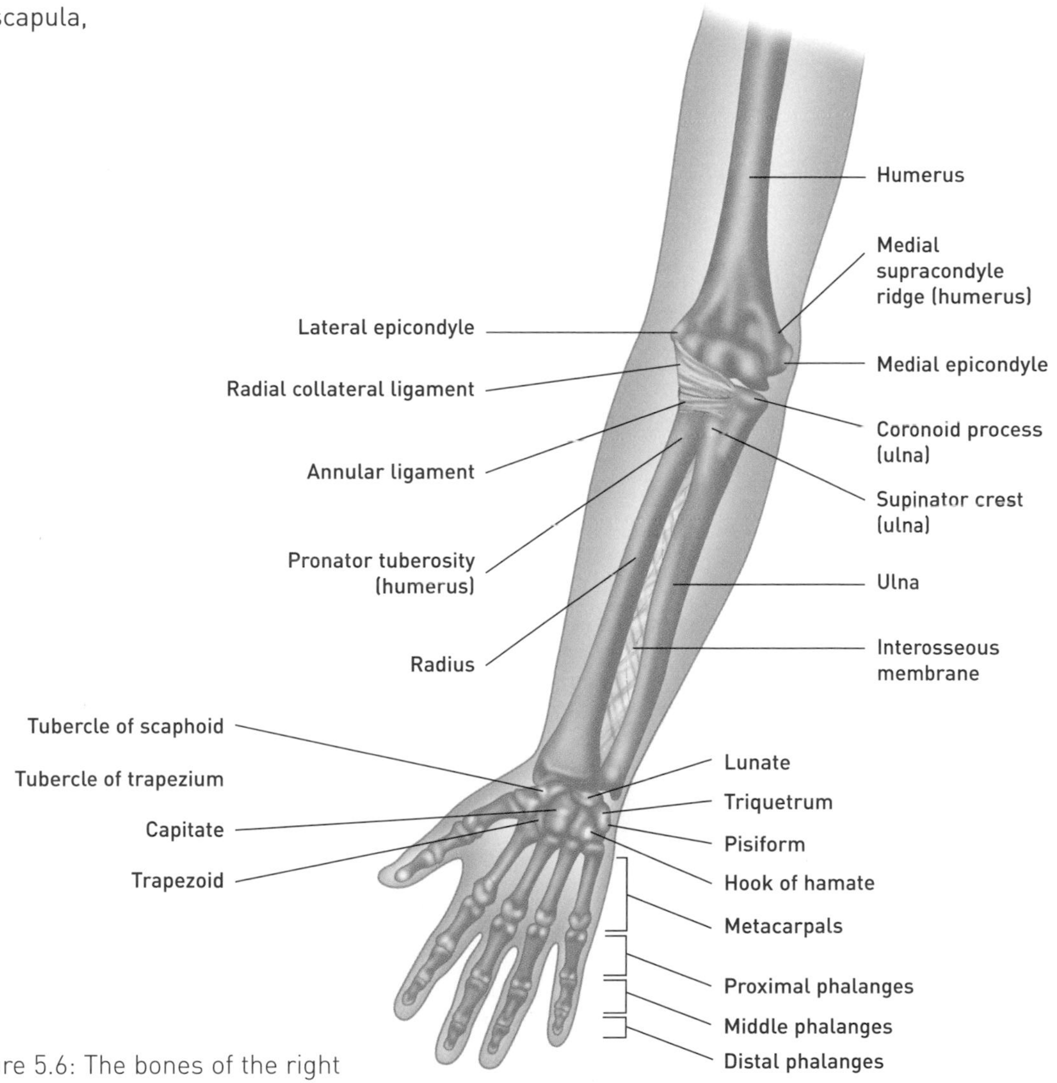

Clavicle (cut)
Acromion
Coracoid process
Glenoid fossa
Lateral border
Scapula

Figure 5.5: The pectoral girdle (anterior view).

Humerus
Medial supracondyle ridge (humerus)
Lateral epicondyle
Radial collateral ligament
Medial epicondyle
Annular ligament
Coronoid process (ulna)
Pronator tuberosity (humerus)
Supinator crest (ulna)
Radius
Ulna
Interosseous membrane
Tubercle of scaphoid
Tubercle of trapezium
Lunate
Capitate
Triquetrum
Trapezoid
Pisiform
Hook of hamate
Metacarpals
Proximal phalanges
Middle phalanges
Distal phalanges

Figure 5.6: The bones of the right forearm and hand (anterior view).

Pelvic girdle: attaches leg to skeleton (ilium, ischium, and pubis).

Leg bones: femur, tibia, fibula, patella, tarsals (talus, calcaneus, others), metatarsals, phalanges (distal, middle, proximal).

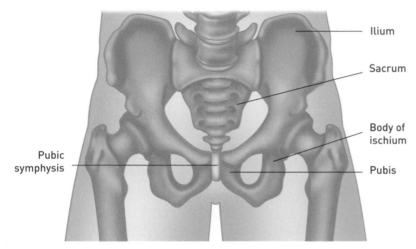

Figure 5.7: The pelvic girdle.

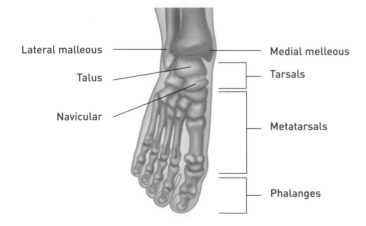

Figure 5.8a: The foot bones.

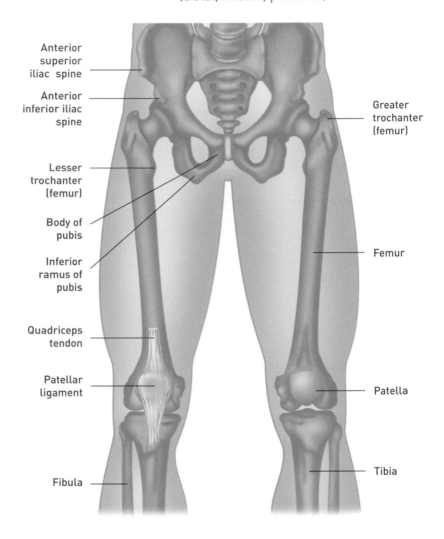

Figure 5.8b: Pelvic girdle to knee (anterior view).

Fractures

Although bones are rigid, they do bend to a certain degree to allow force to be absorbed through the body. Once a bone is bent passed this point, it will crack or break. This crack or break is known as a *fracture*. When a bone has been broken and then set, it undergoes *calcification*, which is the laying down of new bone to repair the damage. The break is initially splinted by fibrocartilage, which is later replaced by bone. Initially, an excess of bone is laid down, but this reduces over several months, so that a properly set, broken bone will return to almost as good as new.

Types of Fracture

CLOSED   A closed fracture occurs when a bone is broken or cracked.

OPEN   An open fracture occurs when a bone breaks and extends out through the skin.

COMPLICATED A complicated fracture occurs when a bone breaks and causes internal damage to tissues or organs.

PATHOLOGICAL Pathological fractures occur due to a disease in the bone.

STRESS   Stress fractures occur due to overuse of a bone causing a tiny crack to form at the site. These fractures are the most common in the sporting industry and usually occur when there is an increase in intensity in training or change of activity. They can also occur due to surface changing (e.g. a cross-country runner changing to road running) and are common if bad footwear is worn for shock absorption. Female athletes are more prone to stress fractures for many medical reasons. The most common site of these fractures would be the weight-bearing bones in the lower leg.

a.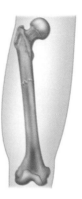

b.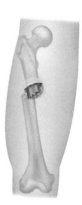

c.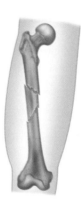

d.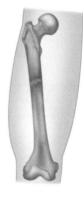

e.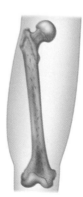

Figure 5.9: Types of fracture; a) closed, b) open, c) complicated, d) pathological, e) stress.

Causes of a Fracture

DIRECT FORCE   Force is applied sufficiently to cause the bone to fracture at the site of impact.

INDIRECT FORCE   Force is applied to one end of the bone (entrance) and the force is transmitted up the limb or body causing the exit bones to fracture, e.g. a fall from a height, the shock enters the body at the feet. The force will travel up and exit the body at the shoulders causing them to fracture.

SPASM-INDUCED   Due to severe overstretching of a limb or to acute muscle spasm which causes the bone to bend past its normal limitations. For example, a common cause of this injury would be a player mis-kicking a ball sending his leg into a violent over-extension.

Signs and Symptoms of a Closed Fracture

- Pain
- Tender to touch at the site of the fracture
- Redness of area – bruising
- Swelling will develop
- Loss of movement
- Irregularity – shortening of a limb
- Crepitus may be heard – grating of bone ends
- May have heard snapping sound
- Shock

Signs and Symptoms of an Open Fracture

- Pain
- Bone end will be visible
- Lacerated wound with bleeding
- Tender to touch at the site of the fracture
- Redness of area – bruising
- Swelling will develop
- Loss of movement
- Irregularity – shortening of a limb
- Crepitus may be heard – grating of bone ends
- May have heard snapping sound
- Shock

Signs and Symptoms of a Complicated Fracture

- Pain
- Tender to touch at the site of the fracture
- Redness of area – bruising
- Swelling will develop
- Loss of movement
- Irregularity – shortening of a limb
- Signs and symptoms of internal bleeding (depending on area of injury), e.g. ribcage – bleeding when coughing; pelvis – bleeding in urine
- Crepitus may be heard – grating of bone ends
- May have heard snapping sound
- Shock

Signs and Symptoms of a Pathological Fracture

- History of bone disease (brittle bone, osteoporosis)
- Pain

- Tender to touch at the site of the fracture
- Redness of area – bruising
- Swelling will develop
- Loss of movement
- Irregularity – shortening of a limb
- Crepitus may be heard – grating of bone ends
- May have heard snapping sound
- Shock

Signs and Symptoms of a Stress Fracture

- History of the problem, change of activity
- Pain on weight-bearing or increase of activity
- Tender to touch at the site of the fracture
- Redness of area – bruising
- Swelling may develop
- Reduction in the range of movement
- Shock

Principles of Treating Closed, Stress and Pathological Fractures

- Place a cold compress on the site (necrosis will occur if using ice wrap with cloth or tissue)
- Apply gentle traction to the injured limb
- Immobilize with SAM® Splint and bandages
- Treat for shock
- Arrange for transport to hospital

Principles of Treating Open Fractures

- Place a sterile dressing over the wound site
- Place roller bandages and padding either side of the visible bone end
- Secure another roller bandage around the padding and dressing (be careful not to press on the bone end, use additional padding to rise above the bone end where necessary)
- Immobilize with SAM® Splint and bandages inferior and superior to the fracture site (do not move the limb if the patient finds it painful, treat fracture in position of impact)
- Check the circulation of the injured limb (arm – capillary refill / leg – distal pulse)
- If bleeding persists, apply further padding and secure with roller bandage (never remove initial bandaging)
- Treat for shock
- Arrange for transport to hospital

Principles of Treating Complicated Fractures

- Treatment varies depending on the fracture site area
- Call for an ambulance
- Treat for shock
- Immobilize injured area
- Place a cold compress on the site (necrosis will occur if using ice wrap with cloth or tissue)
- Place the patient lying down in a comfortable position
- Maintain an open airway
- Be prepared to resuscitate
- Treat shock

Risk Factors of Uncontrolled Movement of Fractures

- Pain will be increased therefore increasing level of shock
- Loss of the patient's trust (it is vital to ensure that this trust is maintained at all times)
- Rupture or tear internal tissues (slowing the healing process)
- Rupture or tear blood vessels, nerves or organs
- Cause bone to protrude through the skin (a closed fracture becomes an open fracture)

- Cause bone to impale a vital organ (a close fracture becomes a complicated fracture)
- Cause internal bleeding
- Increase healing time

Treatment and Bandaging of Closed Fractures to the Skull

- Lie the patient down
- Examine the eyes and ears to rule out damage or injury to the brain
- If bleeding or straw coloured fluid is present, treat as a compression
- Examine the nose and mouth for bleeding
- Apply ice to injury site
- Place the patient in the recovery position on the injured side
- Call for an ambulance
- Treat for shock
- Monitor vital signs

Treatment and Bandaging of Closed Fractures to the Face

- Lie the patient down
- Examine the eyes and ears to rule out damage or injury to the brain
- Examine the nose and mouth for bleeding
- Apply ice to injury site
- Call for an ambulance
- Treat for shock
- Monitor vital signs

Treatment and Bandaging of Closed Fractures to the Neck
(*see* spinal injuries)

Treatment and Bandaging of Closed Fractures to the Back
(*see* spinal injuries)

Treatment and Bandaging of Closed Fractures to the Shoulders

- Lie the patient down
- Examine the shoulder
- Apply ice to the injury site

If the patient can move their arm, place the injured arm in an elevation sling:

- Tie a broad fold bandage around the elbow and torso to support the limb
- Refer to hospital
- Treat for shock
- Monitor vital signs

If the patient cannot move the arm, glide the arm gently into line with the torso. Using the natural hollows of the body (neck, and lumbar spine regions), place 3 broad folds under the patient. Place:

  (i) Mid humerus point (upper arm)
  (ii) Elbow point
  (iii) Lower radius (wrist) point

- Tie the broad folds on the uninjured side of the torso
- Refer to hospital
- Treat for shock
- Monitor vital signs

Treatment and Bandaging of Closed Fractures to the Upper Arm

- Lie the patient down
- Examine the arm
- Apply ice to the injury site

If the patient can move their arm, place the injured arm in a large arm sling:

- Refer to hospital
- Treat for shock
- Monitor vital signs

If the patient cannot move the arm, glide the arm gently into line with the torso. Using the natural hollows of the body (neck, and lumbar spine regions), place 3 broad folds under the patient. Place:

    (i) Superior to the fracture site

    (ii) Inferior to the fracture site

    (iii) Lower radius (wrist) point

- Tie the broad folds on the uninjured side of the torso
- Refer to hospital
- Treat for shock
- Monitor vital signs

Treatment and Bandaging of Closed Fractures to the Lower Arm

- Lie the patient down
- Examine the arm
- Apply ice to the injury site

If the patient can move their arm, place the injured arm in a large arm sling:

- Refer to hospital
- Treat for shock
- Monitor vital signs

If the patient cannot move the arm, glide the arm gently into line with the torso. Using the natural hollows of the body (neck, and lumbar spine regions), place 3 broad folds under the patient. Place:

    (i) Superior to the fracture site

    (ii) Inferior to the fracture site

    (iii) Lower radius (wrist) point

- Tie the broad folds on the uninjured side of the torso
- Refer to hospital
- Treat for shock
- Monitor vital signs

Treatment and Bandaging of Closed Fractures to the Hand

- Lie the patient down
- Examine the hand
- Apply ice to the injury site
- Place the injured hand in a large arm sling
- Treat for shock
- Monitor vital signs
- Refer to hospital

Treatment and Bandaging of Closed Fractures to the Ribs and Sternum

- Lie the patient down
- Examine the ribcage and sternum
- Apply ice to the injury site
- Incline the patient towards the injured side
- Place the arm on the injured side in an elevation sling
- Refer to hospital
- Treat for shock
- Monitor vital signs

Treatment and Bandaging of Closed Fractures to the Pelvis

- Lie the patient down
- Examine the pelvis
- Check for rectal, penal or vaginal discharge or bleeding (indications of internal bleeding)
- If discharge is present, apply padding to the area to facilitate drainage
- If bleeding is present, apply padding and secure with broad fold bandage to control the bleeding
- Apply a figure of 8 bandage to the ankles
- Apply broad fold bandage to the knees
- Bend the knees (approx. 20 degrees) and place blankets under to support
- Call for an ambulance
- Treat for shock
- Monitor vital signs

Treatment and Bandaging of Closed Fractures to the Upper Leg

- Lie the patient down
- Examine the injured site
- Apply ice to the fracture site

Using the natural hollows of the body (ankles, knees, and inferior buttocks), place 5 broad fold bandages under the patient. Place:

    (i) Under the ankles

    (ii) Superior to the fracture site

    (iii) Inferior to the fracture site

    (iv) Under the knees

    (v) Mid tibial region

- Place padding between the knees and ankles
- Gently glide the legs together (move the uninjured to injured)
- Tie a figure of 8 bandage to the ankles first
- Tie superior next
- Tie off the remaining bandages
- All bandages should be tied on the uninjured side
- Apply broad fold bandage to the knees
- Call for an ambulance
- Treat for shock
- Monitor vital signs

Treatment and Bandaging of Closed Fractures to the Lower Leg

- Lie the patient down
- Examine the injured site
- Apply ice to the fracture site

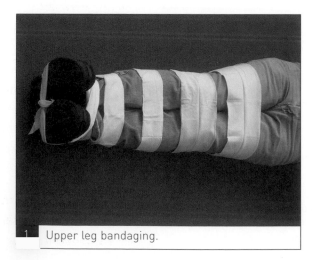

1   Upper leg bandaging.

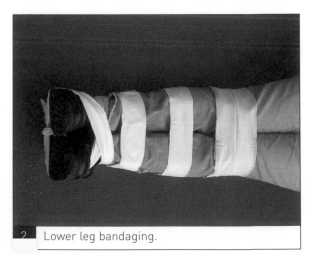

2   Lower leg bandaging.

Using the natural hollows of the body (ankles, knees, and inferior buttocks), place 5 broad fold bandages under the patient. Place:

(i) Under the ankles

(ii) Superior to the fracture site

(iii) Inferior to the fracture site

(iv) Under the knees

(v) Mid femoral region

• Place padding between the knees and ankles
• Gently glide the legs together (move the uninjured to injured)
• Tie a figure of 8 bandage to the ankles first
• Tie superior next
• Tie off the remaining bandages
• All bandages should be tied on the uninjured side
• Apply broad fold bandage to the knees
• Call for an ambulance
• Treat for shock
• Monitor vital signs

Treatment and Bandaging of Closed Fractures to the Knee

• Lie the patient down
• Examine the knee

If the patient can move the knee:

• Bend the knee (approx. 20 degrees) and place blankets under to support

If the patient cannot bend the knee, using the natural hollows of the body (ankles, knees, and inferior buttocks), place 5 broad fold bandages under the patient. Place:

(i) Under the ankles

(ii) Superior to the fracture site

(iii) Inferior to the fracture site

(iv) Mid tibial region

(v) Mid femoral region

• Place padding between the knees and ankles
• Gently glide the legs together (move the uninjured to injured)
• Tie a figure of 8 bandage to the ankles first
• Tie superior next
• Tie off the remaining bandages
• Call for an ambulance
• Treat for shock
• Monitor vital signs

Treatment and Bandaging of Closed Fractures to the Ankle and Foot

• Lie the patient down
• Examine the injured site
• Apply ice to the fracture site

Using the natural hollows of the body (ankles, knees, and inferior buttocks), place 4 broad fold bandages under the patient. Place:

(i) Under the ankles to be tied around the toes

(ii) Superior to the fracture site

(iii) Inferior to the fracture site

(iv) Under the knees

• Place padding between the knees and ankles
• Gently glide the legs together (move the uninjured to injured)
• Tie a figure of 8 bandage to the ankles first
• Tie superior next

- Tie off the remaining bandages
- All bandages should be tied on the uninjured side
- Apply broad fold bandage to the knees
- Call for an ambulance
- Treat for shock
- Monitor vital signs

Treatment and Bandaging of Open Fractures to the Skull

- Lie the patient down
- Examine the eyes and ears to rule out damage or injury to the brain
- If bleeding or straw coloured fluid is present, treat as compression
- Examine the nose and mouth for bleeding
- Place a sterile dressing over the wound site
- Place roller bandages and padding either side of the visible bone end
- Secure another roller bandage around the padding and dressing (be careful not to press on the bone end; use additional padding to rise above the bone end where necessary)
- Place the patient in the recovery position on the injured side
- Call for an ambulance
- Treat for shock
- Monitor vital signs

Treatment and Bandaging of Open Fractures to the Face

- Lie the patient down
- Examine the eyes and ears to rule out damage or injury to the brain
- Examine the nose and mouth for bleeding
- Place a sterile dressing over the wound site
- Place roller bandages and padding either side of the visible bone end
- Secure another roller bandage around the padding and dressing (be careful not to press on the bone end; use additional padding to rise above the bone end where necessary)

- Call for an ambulance
- Treat for shock
- Monitor vital signs

Treatment and Bandaging of Open Fractures to the Neck
(*see* spinal injuries)

Treatment and Bandaging of Open Fractures to the Back
(*see* spinal injuries)

Treatment and Bandaging of Open Fractures to the Shoulders

- Lie the patient down
- Examine the shoulder
- Place a sterile dressing over the wound site
- Place roller bandages and padding either side of the visible bone end
- Secure another roller bandage around the padding and dressing (be careful not to press on the bone end; use additional padding to rise above the bone end where necessary)

If the patient can move their arm, place the injured arm in an elevation sling:

- Tie a broad fold bandage around the elbow and torso to support the limb
- Refer to hospital
- Treat for shock
- Monitor vital signs

If the patient cannot move the arm, glide the arm gently into line with the torso. Using the natural hollows of the body (neck, and lumbar spine regions) place 3 broad folds under the patient. Place:

(i) Mid humerus point (upper arm)
(ii) Elbow point
(iii) Lower radius (wrist) point

- Tie the broad folds on the uninjured side of the torso
- Refer to hospital
- Treat for shock
- Monitor vital signs

Treatment and Bandaging of Open Fractures to the Upper Arm

- Lie the patient down
- Examine the arm
- Place a sterile dressing over the wound site
- Place roller bandages and padding either side of the visible bone end
- Secure another roller bandage around the padding and dressing (be careful not to press on the bone end; use additional padding to rise above the bone end where necessary)

If the patient can move their arm, place the injured arm in a large arm sling:

- Refer to hospital
- Treat for shock
- Monitor vital signs

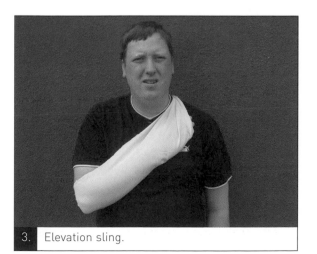

3. Elevation sling.

If the patient cannot move the arm, glide the arm gently into line with the torso. Using the natural hollows of the body (neck, and lumbar spine regions), place 3 broad folds under the patient. Place:

(i) Superior to the fracture site

(ii) Inferior to the fracture site

(iii) Lower radius (wrist) point

- Tie the broad folds on the uninjured side of the torso
- Refer to hospital
- Treat for shock
- Monitor vital signs

Treatment and Bandaging of Open Fractures to the Lower Arm

- Lie the patient down
- Examine the arm
- Place a sterile dressing over the wound site
- Place roller bandages and padding either side of the visible bone end
- Secure another roller bandage around the padding and dressing (be careful not to press on the bone end; use additional padding to rise above the bone end where necessary)

If the patient can move their arm, place the injured arm in a large arm sling:

- Refer to hospital
- Treat for shock
- Monitor vital signs

If the patient cannot move the arm, glide the arm gently into line with the torso. Using the natural hollows of the body (neck, and lumbar spine regions) place 3 broad folds under the patient. Place:

(i) Superior to the fracture site

(ii) Inferior to the fracture site

(iii) Lower radius (wrist) point

- Tie the broad folds on the uninjured side of the torso
- Refer to hospital
- Treat for shock
- Monitor vital signs

Treatment and Bandaging of Open Fractures to the Hand

- Lie the patient down
- Examine the hand
- Place a sterile dressing over the wound site
- Place roller bandages and padding either side of the visible bone end
- Secure another roller bandage around the padding and dressing (be careful not to press on the bone end; use additional padding to rise above the bone end where necessary)
- Place the injured hand in a large arm sling
- Treat for shock
- Monitor vital signs
- Refer to hospital

Treatment and Bandaging of Open Fractures to the Ribs and Sternum

- Lie the patient down
- Examine the ribcage and sternum
- Place a sterile dressing over the wound site
- Place roller bandages and padding either side of the visible bone end
- Secure another roller bandage around the padding and dressing (be careful not to press on the bone end; use additional padding to rise above the bone end where necessary)
- Incline the patient towards the injured side
- Place the arm on the injured side in an elevation sling
- Refer to hospital
- Treat for shock
- Monitor vital signs

Treatment and Bandaging of Open Fractures to the Pelvis

- Lie the patient down
- Examine the pelvis
- Check for rectal, penal or vaginal discharge or bleeding (indications of internal bleeding)
- If discharge is present, apply padding to the area to facilitate drainage
- If bleeding is present, apply padding and secure with broad fold bandage to control bleeding
- Place a sterile dressing over the wound site
- Place roller bandages and padding either side of the visible bone end
- Secure another roller bandage around the padding and dressing (be careful not to press on the bone end; use additional padding to rise above the bone end where necessary)
- Apply a figure of 8 bandage to the ankles
- Apply broad fold bandage to the knees
- Bend the knees (approx. 20 degrees) and place blankets under to support
- Call for an ambulance
- Treat for shock
- Monitor vital signs

Treatment and Bandaging of Open Fractures to the Upper Leg

- Lie the patient down
- Examine the injured site
- Place a sterile dressing over the wound site
- Place roller bandages and padding either side of the visible bone end
- Secure another roller bandage around the padding and dressing (be careful not to press on the bone end; use additional padding to rise above the bone end where necessary)

Using the natural hollows of the body (ankles, knees, and inferior buttocks), place 5 broad fold bandages under the patient. Place:

(i) Under the ankles

(ii) Superior to the fracture site

(iii) Inferior to the fracture site

(iv) Under the knees

(v) Mid tibial region

- Place padding between the knees and ankles
- Gently glide the legs together (move the uninjured to injured)
- Tie a figure of 8 bandage to the ankles first
- Tie superior next
- Tie off the remaining bandages
- All bandages should be tied on the uninjured side
- Apply broad fold bandage to the knees
- Call for an ambulance
- Treat for shock
- Monitor vital signs

Treatment and Bandaging of Open Fractures to the Lower Leg

- Lie the patient down
- Examine the injured site
- Place a sterile dressing over the wound site
- Place roller bandages and padding either side of the visible bone end
- Secure another roller bandage around the padding and dressing (be careful not to press on the bone end, use additional padding to rise above the bone end where necessary)

Using the natural hollows of the body (ankles, knees, and inferior buttocks), place 5 broad fold bandages under the patient:

(i) Under the ankles

(ii) Superior to the fracture site

(iii) Inferior to the fracture site

(iv) Under the knees

(v) Mid femoral region

- Place padding between the knees and ankles
- Gently glide the legs together (move the uninjured to injured)
- Tie a figure of 8 bandage to the ankles first
- Tie superior next
- Tie off remaining bandages
- All bandages should be tied on the uninjured side
- Apply a broad fold bandage to the knees
- Call for an ambulance
- Treat for shock
- Monitor vital signs

Treatment and Bandaging of Open Fractures to the Knee

- Lie the patient down
- Examine the knee
- Place a sterile dressing over the wound site
- Place roller bandages and padding either side of the visible bone end
- Secure another roller bandage around the padding and dressing (be careful not to press on the bone end; use additional padding to rise above the bone end where necessary)

Using the natural hollows of the body (ankles, knees, and inferior buttocks), place 5 broad fold bandages under the patient. Place:

(i) Under the ankles

(ii) Superior to the fracture site

(iii) Inferior to the fracture site

(iv) Mid tibial region

(v) Mid femoral region

- Place padding between the knees and ankles
- Gently glide the legs together (move the uninjured to injured)
- Tie a figure of 8 bandage to the ankles first
- Tie superior next
- Tie off the remaining bandages
- Call for an ambulance
- Treat for shock
- Monitor vital signs

Treatment and Bandaging of Open Fractures to the Ankle and Foot

- Lie the patient down
- Examine the injured site
- Place a sterile dressing over the wound site
- Place roller bandages and padding either side of the visible bone end
- Secure another roller bandage around the padding and dressing (be careful not to press on the bone end; use additional padding to rise above the bone end where necessary)

Using the natural hollows of the body (ankles, knees, and inferior buttocks), place 4 broad fold bandages under the patient. Place:

(i) Under the ankles to be tied around the toes

(ii) Superior to the fracture site

(iii) Inferior to the fracture site

(iv) Under the knees

- Place padding between the knees and ankles
- Gently glide the legs together (move the uninjured to injured)
- Tie a figure of 8 bandage to ankles first
- Tie superior next
- Tie off the remaining bandages
- All bandages should be tied on the uninjured side

- Apply broad fold bandage to the knees
- Call for an ambulance
- Treat for shock
- Monitor vital signs

Treatment and / or Bandaging of Complicated Fractures to the:

Skull:	*see* head injuries	page 90
Face:	*see* head injuries	page 90
Neck:	*see* spinal injuries	page 85
Back:	*see* spinal injuries	page 85
Shoulders:	*see* dislocations and open fractures to the shoulder	pages 68 & 60
Upper arm:	*see* open arm fractures	page 61
Lower arm:	*see* open arm fractures	page 61
Hand:	*see* open arm fractures	page 62
Ribs and sternum:	*see* chest injuries	page 95
Pelvis:	*see* internal bleeding and fractured pelvis	pages 28 & 62
Upper leg:	*see* internal bleeding and leg fractures	pages 28 & 62
Lower leg:	*see* internal bleeding and leg fractures	pages 28 & 63
Knee:	*see* internal bleeding and leg fractures	pages 28 & 63
Ankle and foot:	*see* internal bleeding and leg fractures	pages 28 & 64

6. SAM® Splint

The Story of Seaberg

Dr. Sam Scheinberg, surgeon, inventor of SAM® Splint

In 1968, whilst serving as a trauma surgeon in Vietnam, Dr. Sam Scheinberg observed a number of problems with the available cardboard, wire ladder and air splints. They were bulky, lacked reusability and often caused more harm than good. Years later, after operating 24 hours without rest, Dr. Scheinberg was relaxing watching TV. He was chewing gum and rolling the gum wrapper around his little finger, when he noticed this flimsy material was, to some degree, functioning as a splint. Sam, a methodical orthopaedic surgeon, had an "Ah-Ha" experience. He recognised the splinting properties of the gum wrapper came from its shape. The next day, he and his wife Cherrie obtained a thin piece of aluminium (a large gum wrapper) and coated it with adhesive tape. Thus came into being the first SAM® Splint. This would have been the end of the story had it not been for the high-energy Cherrie, who proceeded to literally chase Sam around the house until he promised to bring the splint to market. Sam likes to say it was the luckiest ten minutes of nagging in his life.

Together, starting in their kitchen, Sam and Cherrie began the Seaberg Company, Inc., manufacturers of the SAM® Splint. In 1985, the first splint was introduced, which was also known as the "Pocket Cast". Today, the SAM® Splint is one of the most popular emergency splints in the world.

Truly the standard for pre-hospital and wilderness care. Today's SAM® Splint is more or less an enlarged version of Dr. Scheinberg's original 'gum wrapper' splint. The standard size is 36 inches (91 cm) long and weighs only 4 ounces (113 grams). Its light weight and flexibility easily allows you to fold or shape the splint to fit in any kit.

Section One:
SAM® Splint Basic Instructions and General Information

The SAM® Splint is a long rectangle of "zero temper," very thin aluminium alloy sandwiched between two layers of high quality dermatological safe ethylene vinyl acetate closed pore foam. It is available in the following sizes:

Standard size:	The most commonly used size suitable for adults and children. Length is 36 inches (91cm), width 4.25 inches (10.6cm), depth 0.25 inches (.6cm), weight 4 ounces (113 grams).
Junior size:	Useful for adult upper extremities, adult ankles when used in pairs, and in children upper and lower extremity injuries. Length is 18 inches (46cm), width 4.25 inches (10.6cm), depth 0.25 inches (.6cm), weight 2 ounces (56 grams).
Wrist splint:	Used for wrist support or for IV boards. Length is 9 inches (22.5 cm), width 4.25 inches (10.6cm), depth 0.25 inches (.6cm), weight 1 ounce (28 grams).
Finger splint:	Useful for finger splints, neonatal IV boards, or shoe inserts. Length is 4.25 inches (10.6cm), width 2 inches (5cm), depth 0.25 inches (.6cm), the weight .10 ounce (2.8 grams).

A SAM® Splint in its virgin state (without any bends) is completely malleable. When a curve or fold is placed anywhere across its longitudinal axis, it becomes rigid and suitable for splinting. Secondary reverse curves placed along the edges dramatically increase the splint's strength. A "T" bend produces exceptional rigidity.

The SAM® Splint is radiolucent, almost invisible on X-ray. It should not be removed for radiographs. It is designed to function through the extreme ranges of normal ambient temperatures. It is waterproof, but not fireproof.

The closed pore EVA foam will not flash when exposed to flames but will begin to melt and eventually ignite after approximately 8 seconds.

The SAM® Splint is easily cut with ordinary scissors. Trauma shears are not required. Cutting exposes the thin aluminium core. Unless serrated scissors have been used, the aluminium is usually not very sharp. To prevent any injury from the exposed edge, we recommend folding the edge on itself 1 to 2 times. Covering the edge with tape is also effective.

The foam used in the SAM® Splint was selected for its "cleanability". Whether cut or used intact, the splint can be cleaned with antiseptic soap and water or with almost any protocol cleaning solution. I prefer a hypochlorite cleaning solution, in an inexpensive 1:9 mixture of commercially available bleach and water.

The closed pore foam, which promotes effective cleaning, does not however absorb or allow passage of air or perspiration. This does not present a problem during short-term use. If however the splint is to be maintained for prolonged periods (hours to days), some absorbent material such as cotton cloth, case padding, or double tubular stockinette should be placed between the splint and patient to prevent skin maceration and odour.

Although the EVA foam does provide some padding, when prolonged use is contemplated, additional soft padding should be placed around all bony prominences to prevent pressure points.

Section Two:
SAM® Splint User Instructions–Upper Extremity

Finger

- The commercially available SAM® Finger Splint (or a similar size piece cut from a larger splint) can be used with a single longitudinal bend
- Bend the splint into a semi-circle for strength
- Squeeze the ends of the splint together to create a fingertip guard

If you prefer to splint the finger in a curved functional position, fold one edge of the splint down upon itself and the opposite edge up at a right angle. You will then be able to curve the splint as needed. Note: use your own finger as a template before applying to an injured patient.

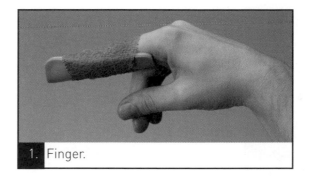

1. Finger.

Thumb (carpal bone)

For splinting the thumb, or in the case of a suspected carpal bone fracture or dislocation, a commercially available wrist SAM® Splint or an appropriately sized piece cut from a larger splint is first moulded around you own wrist and thumb in the shape of a thumb Spica. The thumb section is then maintained with your wrap of choice (tape, gauze, or elastic wrap). The splint is then applied to the patient and secured with elastic wrap.

Wrist Splint

A volar wrist splint for simple sprains, night splints, or carpal tunnel splints is also first shaped to your own wrist before applying to the patient. The splint is typically moulded in the "cock-up" functional position. This position is secured and the splint strengthened by bending up its ulnar border. For prolonged use (more than a few hours), cover the splint with absorbent cloth such as cotton. I typically use double-layered tubular stockinet and secure the splint with an elastic wrap.

Distal Radio-ulnar Joint (Wrist) Fractures

Option 1:   The classic "sugar-tong" configuration provides support of the distal radius and ulna, and to some extent, prevent rotation. First, fold the standard size SAM® Splint in half to create two equal limbs. Then, beginning at the end of one limb, use your thumbs to produce a gentle cross-sectional curve of a semi-circle. The curve can be quickly deepened, by squeezing. Do not extend the curve all the way down the limb, as this will limit your ability to mould the "sugar-tong" around the elbow. After completing the bends in the first limb, create a similar curve in the opposite limb. Fold the splint around the elbow and secure to the extremity with your wrap of choice. Excess splint should be folded back to allow good visualisation of the fingers.

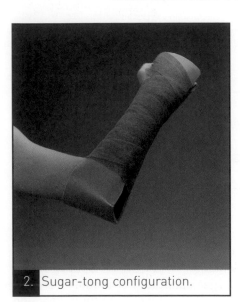

2. Sugar-tong configuration.

Option 2:   The "double layer" configuration. A double layered splint is created, by folding the standard size SAM® Splint in half upon itself. This two-layered splint is then curved into a cross-sectional half-circle and moulded to your own extremity. Small adjustments are made after applying the splint to the patient.

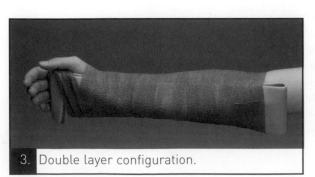

3. Double layer configuration.

Option 3:   The "T-bend" configuration. This configuration is exceptionally strong. The standard size SAM® Splint is first folded in half creating two limbs. One limb is folded on itself along its longitudinal axis. The edges of the fold are then bent in a contrary direction to create a T-shaped beam. This T-beam is then placed as a support against the opposite limb, which is curved to fit the extremity.

Forearm, Radius and Ulna, Midshaft Fractures

The "sugar-tong" configuration is preferred, but "double layered" and "T-bend" configurations can also be used.

Proximal Radio-ulnar Joint Fractures or Dislocations

The "sugar-tong" configuration supported by a sling is recommended.

Elbow Dislocations

Typically in an elbow dislocation, the upper extremity is swollen, has an irregular contour, and is lying in the extended position. In this situation, splint the extremity as it lies. Do not try to force the dislocated elbow into a flexed position. First create the proper splint length by measuring a section of a standard size SAM® Splint extending from just below the patient's axilla to the fingertips. Fold over any excess splint. Next,

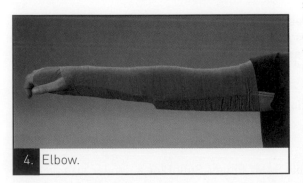

4. Elbow.

contour a cross-sectional curve or semi-circle down the entire measured length of the splint. Apply the SAM® Splint from just below the axilla to the fingertips and secure with your wrap of choice.

Humeral Shaft (Upper Arm) Fractures

When the humeral shaft fracture is displaced, the upper arm is typically shortened and swollen. To splint this fracture, fold the standard size SAM® Splint on itself to create a 9 inch (23cm) section of double-layered splint. Then fold this double layer into a hook shape. With the elbows in the flexed position, place this hook around the elbow and arm as illustrated.

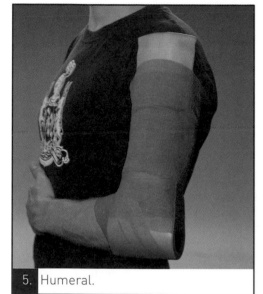

5. Humeral.

Contour a semi-circle cross section portion in the splint extending up the lateral aspect of the arm and secure the splint to the arm with your wrap of choice. You may fold any excess over the shoulder or back upon itself. Apply sling and swath.

Humeral Head and Neck (Shoulder) Fractures

A sling and swath or "Velpeau" dressing is recommended. No splint is required.

Anterior Dislocation of the Shoulder

In this common dislocation, the patient's arm is typically most comfortable when supported in the abducted (sitting away from the body) position. The arm can be supported in this manner with a rolled blanket, ski parka, pillow or SAM® Splint "triangle". To create a "triangle" your splint is first folded into thirds. This produces three equal 9 inch (23cm) sections of splints.

Fold the outer sections along the longitudinal axis, leaving the middle section flat. Hook the outer folded ends together, producing a triangle. A more rounded gentler curve or semi-circle is then folded along the longitudinal axis of the middle section of the splint. This curve, however, is made in the opposite direction.

The triangle is then placed in the axilla and used to support the abducted arm. The arm triangle is held in place by the patient or secured to the patient's trunk with your wrap of choice.

Section Three:
SAM® Splint User Instructions–Lower Extremity

Fractured or Sprained Ankle with Deformity

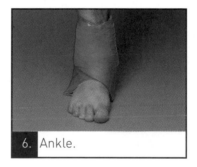

6. Ankle.

Based on your protocol, you may choose to splint the ankle as it lies, or apply traction to reduce the deformity. If you are in a remote situation where no assistance is available, an attempt should be made to reduce the deformity. If the deformity persists, fold your splint in a zigzag fashion to approximate the shape of the deformed extremity.

Curve the splint in cross-section to create rigidity, pad and apply the splint. Support the splint with a second splint, curved for strength. Secure with a wrap.

Fractured or Sprained Ankle with Minimal Deformity

Use the sugar-tong technique as for a wrist fracture but apply to the ankle as a stirrup. Remember to apply padding just above and around the bony prominences (malleoli). Secure with your wrap of choice.

A "Figure I" splint can also be used for the ankle especially when weight-bearing may be required. Again remember to apply padding just above and around the malleoli.

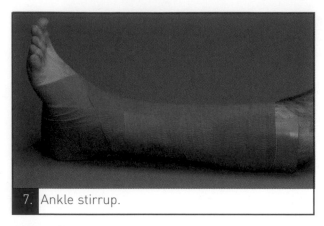

7. Ankle stirrup.

Lower Tibial Shaft Fractures

A fracture located at the lower end of the tibia, just above the ankle, can be treated like an ankle sprain or fracture and splinted with a sugar-tong stirrup. A "stirrup" splint can be used in combination with a "Figure 8" splint for greater stability.

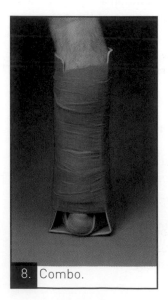

8. Combo.

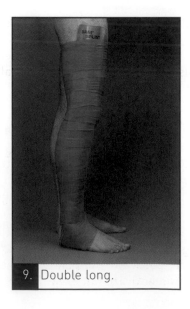

9. Double long.

Mid and Upper Tibial Shaft Fractures

In a fracture located higher up the tibial shaft, the knee and ankle must be immobilised. This is accomplished by using two splints to create a long sugar-tong stirrup. The ends of these splints are folded to create foot-plates which help interlock the two splints together. Note: this technique can also be used for a knee injury.

Knee Injuries

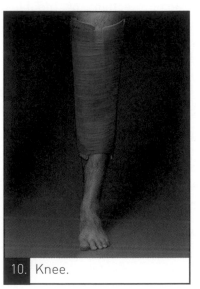

10. Knee.

A standard size SAM® Splint is folded in the centre to form two limbs. The inner edge of one limb is then placed adjacent to and slightly overlapping the inner edge of the opposing limb.

This produces a fan-shaped splint, wider at the top and narrow at the bottom (as the thigh is wider than the calf). The "fan" splint is then secured with tape at the top, middle and bottom. A gentle cross-sectional curve is then moulded into the "fan" splint to contour to the thigh and calf.

Fold a second splint in the same fan-shaped manner. Secure a splint to each side of the knee with your wrap of choice.

Note: This same technique can be used to create an extra wide splint for use on large arms or legs.

Femoral Fractures

The 'sugar-tong stirrup' technique can be used in small children with lower femoral shaft fractures. Otherwise, the SAM® Splint is not appropriate for femoral fractures.

Section Four:
SAM® Splint User Instructions–Neck

Always use your pre-formed "protocol" C-collar. If, however, no such C-collar is available or will not fit, then consider using alternative methods such as a rolled blanket, newspaper, or a SAM® Splint.

Adjustable C-Collar–4 Poster

Fold a standard size SAM® Splint approximately 4 inches (10cm) from one end. Pull the upper edge of this 4-inch section forward to create a round comfortable support for the chin and lower jaw. When you complete this bend, the 4 inch (10cm) section is in a "V" shape and will resemble a pre-formed C-collar. Place this section beneath the chin, taking care to avoid any pressure on the front of the neck.

Next, loop the remaining portion of the splint loosely in a clockwise fashion around the neck and bring the end of the splint down in an oblique direction until it hits the chest. This will give a correct "chin-chest" distance for the front post.

After obtaining the correct chin-chest distance, complete the circle and front post by pushing the end of the splint further around in a clockwise direction. The front post can be deepened by squeezing. Next, insert your index fingers in each side of the looped splint. Pull outward and squeeze to create a snug fit and supporting side posts. When the patient is sitting, a back post can be created in a similar manner. Secure with tape.

Head Bed

If a pre-formed Head Bed is not available, a SAM® Splint can be placed flat beneath the head and then contoured to each side of the head. The remaining ends of the splint are folded into triangles, which apply pressure to each side of the head. These triangles and the head itself are secured with tape.

Section Five:
SAM® Splint User Instructions–Chest / Low Back / Pelvis

Chest–Rib Fractures

Place a standard size SAM® Splint within a 5–6ft (1.5m–1.8m) section of tubular stockinet. Centre the splint in the stockinet so that 1–2 ft (30cm–60cm) of stockinet remains loose on each end. Wrap the stockinet-covered splint around the injured chest area and secure by tying the ends.

Low Back Fractures

Directions as above.

Pelvis Fractures

Directions as above, but should be tied tightly around the padded pelvic rim to help close any open book fracture.

Section 6:
SAM® Splint User Instructions–Alternative Uses

Over the years, many individuals in the emergency medicine and wilderness medicine arenas have developed interesting alternative uses for the SAM® Splint. We have listed a few:

Thomas Half-ring Splint

First create the "foot support" by cutting an 8 inch (20cm) section from an old ski pole. Drill 2 holes, 6 inches (15cm) apart through this foot support section. The hole should be sized, with a larger entry hole and a smaller exit hole to tightly accommodate the tapered end of the ski pole.

Keep the "foot support" section in your pack along with duct tape, safety pins, and strong cord (to be used for traction as desired). To create the 'half-ring, hip support', place two ski poles, handle facing handle, each on the outer third of a standard size flat SAM® Splint.

Roll each end of the splint tightly around the handles, and secure the splint with duct tape. The rolled middle third of the SAM® Splint is then folded as the ski poles are aligned generally parallel to each other. The position of the ski poles is maintained by firmly fitting the tips of the poles into the tapered holes in the "foot support". The rolled "hip support section" of the SAM® Splint between the two ski pole handles is now contoured to resemble a Thomas half-ring. Duct tape thigh and calf supports are then applied and may be reinforced with cloth or elastic wraps.

Flexible Container (SamPan™)

To create a SamPan™, fold a standard size SAM® Splint into a circle. The opposing ends of the splint may be left open or secured with interlocking bends, paper clips or duct tape. Select a standard plastic bag, sized to your desired use. Place the plastic bag within the splint circle and fold any excess bag over the splint edges. The folded portion of the bag can be left free, rolled over the splint or secured with paper clips. You have now created a flexible basin suitable for many uses including:

- The irrigation of scalp, trunk, and extremity wounds. With the ends of the splint left unfastened, the head and neck easily fit within the plastic bag. The pan can be moulded to any area, even between the legs
- For thawing frost bite in a wilderness setting
- For personal hygiene, one can use the SamPan™ as a wash basin, or for collecting body wastes (i.e. emesis basin, urinal or bedpan)
- For use as a rubbish bin
- In food preparation, or as a serving bowl
- For washing dishes
- For general packing or storing of items in suitcases, cupboards, etc.

(**Note from Dr. Scheinberg:** My special thanks to Brian Horner, survival expert, who created the first SamPan™ on the slopes of Mount Denali, and successfully used it to thaw a frost-bitten foot).

Canoe Paddle

One end of the standard size SAM® Splint is rolled to create a hand grip. The splint extending from that grip is folded to a corrugated cross-section. This corrugation provides extreme strength for the paddle stem. The corrugation, although more relaxed, extends into the paddle blade itself. The handle and stem can be supported with duct tape.

Short Snow Shovel

Same as the canoe paddle, except the EVA foam is cut or burned away from the shovel blade. The outer edges may be acutely folded for additional strength.

Flashlight Holder

Cut a small strip of splint sufficiently long enough to wrap around the stem of your glasses and around your flashlight. This will allow you to use your light hands free. It is excellent for reading in bed.

7. Soft Tissue Injuries

Neuromuscular Therapy (NMT)

John Sharkey, Neuromuscular Therapist and Director of the National Training Centre, Ireland

Neuromuscular Therapy (NMT) is a thorough program of recovery from acute and chronic pain syndromes. NMT utilises specific hands-on manual therapy modalities. This unique and scientific approach to muscular and myofascial pain relief aims to bring about a balance between the musculo-skeletal, myofascial and nervous systems. The neuromuscular therapist or physical therapist is educated in advanced anatomy, kinesiology and biomechanics and is trained to work as a member of a medical multidisciplinary team or in a clinical setting.

In Ireland and the UK, the neuromuscular therapist or physical therapist is recognised as an expert leading the field in treatment of myofascial trigger points. NMT treats Trigger Points (TrP's) by deactivating the hyperirritability in muscle that can strongly modulate central nervous system functions. There are only a few specific conditions where NMT may be contra-indicated. These include large bruises, phlebitis, varicose veins, open wounds, undiagnosed lumps and skin infections.

Table 1. Indications for Neuromuscular Therapy.

- Sports Injuries
- Sprains
- Strains
- Arthritis
- Bursitis
- Carpal Tunnel Syndrome
- Acute Pain
- Dental Occlusion Problems
- Headaches
- Joint Immobility
- Migraines
- Muscle Cramps
- Back Pain
- Neck Pain
- Brachial Plexus Entrapment
- Postural Distortions
- Repetitive Strain Injuries
- Skeletal Pain
- Chronic Pain
- Sciatica
- Spinal Discs Herniation
- Scoliosis
- Whiplash
- TMJ Dysfunction

Neuromuscular Therapy is used to address six elements that cause or contribute to pain:

Ischemia:	Lack of blood supply to soft tissues which causes hypersensitivity to touch
Trigger Points:	Highly irritated nodules in muscles which refer pain in predictable patterns to other parts of the body
Nerve Compression or Entrapment:	Pressure on a nerve by soft tissue, cartilage or bone
Postural Distortion:	Imbalance of the musculo-skeletal system off the saggital, frontal or transverse planes
Biomechanical Dysfunction:	Imbalance resulting in neuromuscular inefficiency and faulty movement patterns
Biochemical Influences:	Poor nutrition can sustain or cause inflammation and pain and contribute to the formation of trigger points

Soft tissue injuries occur when ligaments, tendons or muscles are overstretched or torn.

Inflammation

It is important to understand the process of inflammation in order to explain the symptoms and treatment of soft tissue injuries. A well warmed up muscle will be able to stretch without tearing itself whereas a cold muscle will not have the same ability and will stretch to a point and then tear. When muscle fibres tear, they leak out tissue fluid that begins to accumulate locally near the site of injury. Inflammation is the result of this tissue fluid building up at the site of injury. It will generally present by the area becoming very warm, swelling forming at the site, reddening of the skin and tenderness. This process begins immediately after an injury, but it can take 24–72 hours for enough tissue fluid to build up at the site of injury to cause pain or noticeable swelling in minor cases.

It is important that the simple application of cold therapy is applied as soon as possible. This will help to prevent a significant amount of the tissue fluid accumulating. This in turn will significantly shorten the duration of any injury-related disabilities (e.g. time off from work or athletic duties) and hasten a return back to full function.

Cold Therapy

Cold therapy slows down the blood flow to an injury, which cuts down the swelling and pain. Cold therapy can be applied by an ice pack, gel pack, cold water or cold gel, and should be used right after the injury.

Cold therapy is good for soft tissue injuries that may occur with all sporting events. Cold therapy is also called *ice therapy* in the RICE procedure. Cold packs should be made up from sterile material soaked in ice water. Once warmed up, this material should be re-soaked. Cold packs should be applied to the injury site for about 10–15 minutes at a time, every few hours. If at any time you do use ice, make sure to wrap it and never apply ice directly to skin. This process should be completed over the next 24–48 hours until a neuromuscular therapist or physical therapist may evaluate the injury. Application of cold therapy:

• Treatment should not last for more than 15 minutes
• Skin temperature should be monitored regularly during treatment as freeze burns may occur
• Never apply ice directly to the skin as tissue necrosis may occur
• Electrical cooling pads should only be used by qualified therapists or physiotherapists

Contra-indications

Cold therapy (ice) should not be used (if):

• You have no feeling at the injury site
• You have poor circulation, e.g. diabetes
• You are a haemophiliac
• On open wounds or over stitches

Heat Therapy

Heat therapy has the opposite effect to cold therapy when applied to acute (fresh) injuries. It increases the circulation to the injury site and greatly enhances the tissue swelling, increasing the pain. Heat therapy is good for stiffness and ongoing chronic pain. Heat can be applied by hot water bottle, gel packs heated in water, or hot water baths or hot gels.

Application of heat therapy:

• Treatment should not last for more than 15 minutes
• Skin temperature should be monitored regularly during treatment
• Electrical heating pads should only be used by qualified therapists or physiotherapists

Contra-indications

Heat therapy should not be used (if):

• You have no feeling at the injury site
• There is swelling at the site
• You have poor circulation, e.g. diabetes
• You are a haemophiliac
• On open wounds or over stitches
• You have injuries to the eyes, abdomen or genitalia
• On acute injuries

Prevention of Soft Tissue Injuries

It is so easy to get injured during sporting activities, which may leave you injured for long periods of time. Good practice of safe sport should always be followed, mimimising the risk of injury to athletes. Commonsense can prevent many sport injuries; for the extra few minutes it takes to prepare in comparison to months of being injured. Prevention is better than cure. Always consult your neuromuscular therapist if you are injured before commencing exercise or play. Here are a few helpful tips to get you going:

- You should never lock your knees during play or rest
- Do not twist your knees past their normal range of motion
- Keep your feet flat during warm ups and stretching
- Always use the softest surface available when you exercise
- Wear proper shoes with soft, flexible soles. Wearing good brands will be of no benefit if they do not fit correctly. Wear shoes and socks that fit well
- When you jump, land with your knees bent
- Complete a full warm up session before any exercise or play
- Complete a full cool down session after any exercise or play
- Don't eat or drink large amounts before you exercise
- Never strap a joint without a consultation if you are injured
- Most important of all, if you feel pain STOP what you are doing; do not work through it
- Remember PREVENTION is better than CURE!

Ligaments are taut bands of tissue that connect bone to bone at joints. *Tendons* are fibrous elastic tissues that connect muscle to bone. Skeletal muscles consist of bundles of fibres that are enclosed in a connective tissue sheath.

Types of Soft Tissue Injuries

Sprains

A sprain is a partial or complete tear of a ligament. The joints of the body are supported by ligaments that connect one bone to another. When the ligament is over-stretched or torn, it can result in a partial or full tear of the ligament.

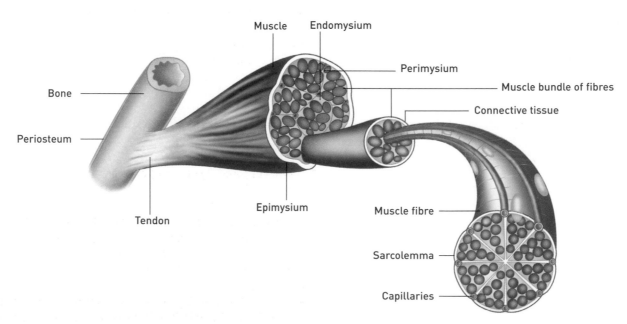

Figure 7.1: Connective tissue sheaths / skeletal muscle.

Signs and Symptoms of a Sprain

- History of the accident (how did the joint receive the impact)
- Pain at the injured joint (e.g. wrist, knee)
- Swelling
- Tender to touch
- Bruising
- Impaired movement at the joint
- Shock

Treatment and Bandaging of a Sprain

- **R** Rest
- **I** Ice (not to be applied directly to the skin, as tissue necrosis will occur)
- **C** Compression bandage to the injured area
- **E** Elevation of the limb
- Immobilize the injured limb, joint
- Treat for shock
- Refer to a doctor
- Refer to hospital if you have any doubt about broken bones

Strains

A strain is the result of an injury to either a muscle or a tendon. The strain may be an over-stretch in the muscle or tendon, or it may be a partial or complete tear in the muscle-and-tendon combination.

Signs and Symptoms of a Strain

- History of the accident (how did the muscle / tendon receive the impact)
- Pain in the muscle or tendon region
- Swelling or visible hollow between the muscle and joint
- Tender to touch
- Bruising
- Impaired movement of the limb
- Shock

Treatment and Bandaging of a Strain

- **R** Rest
- **I** Ice (not to be applied directly to the skin as tissue necrosis will occur)
- **C** Compression bandage to the injured area
- **E** Elevation of the limb
- Immobilize the injured limb, joint
- Treat for shock
- Refer to a neuromuscular therapist
- Refer to hospital if you have any doubt about broken bones

Dislocation

A dislocation is the result of an injury to a joint where one or more bones are displaced from the joint.

Signs and Symptoms of a Dislocation

- History of the accident (how did the joint receive the impact)
- Pain at the joint
- Swelling or visible hollow at the joint
- Tender to touch
- Bruising
- Loss of movement of the limb
- Shock

Treatment and Bandaging of a Dislocation

- **R** Rest
- **I** Ice (not to be applied directly to the skin, as tissue necrosis will occur)
- **C** Compression bandage to the injured area
- **E** Elevation of the limb
- Immobilize the injured limb, joint
- Treat for shock
- Refer to hospital if you have any doubt about broken bones
- NEVER TRY TO RELOCATE (you will cause irreparable damage. This procedure should only be done by a doctor)

Repetitive Strain Injury (RSI)

RSI is the result of continuous overuse of ligaments, muscles or tendons.

Signs and Symptoms of a RSI

• History of the ongoing problem
• Pain at the joint increased with activity
• Swelling
• Tender to touch
• Bruising
• Impaired movement of limb

Treatment and Bandaging of a RSI

• **R** Rest
• **I**   Ice (not to be applied directly to the skin, as tissue necrosis will occur)
• **C** Compression bandage to the injured area
• **E** Elevation of the limb
• Immobilize the injured limb / joint and use a SAM® Splint if you suspect an underlying fracture is present
• Treat for shock
• Refer to a neuromuscular therapist / physical therapist

Cramp

A cramp is an involuntary and forcibly contracted muscle that does not relax. Cramps can affect any muscle under your voluntary control (skeletal muscle). Muscles that span two joints are most prone to cramping. Cramps can involve part or all of a muscle, or several muscles in a group. A cramping muscle may feel hard to the touch and/or appear visibly distorted or twitch beneath the skin. A cramp may last for up to 15 minutes. Pain will vary from slight to acute.

Signs and Symptoms of Cramp

• Sudden intense tightening of a muscle or muscles
• Pain ranging from slight to acute
• Restricted range of motion in the affected joint
• Muscle will be hard to the touch
• Muscle may tear in severe cases

Treatment of Cramp

• Stop doing whatever activity triggered the cramp
• If possible get the patient to contract the opposing muscle to the affected muscle (this will cause the affected muscle to relax)
• Gently stretch and massage the cramping muscle, holding it in a stretched position until the cramp stops
• Apply heat to tense / tight muscles
• Apply cold to sore / tender muscles
• If cramping persists refer to neuromuscular therapist / physical therapist

Common Soft Tissue Injuries Affecting Athletes

Metatarsalgia

This condition is caused by overuse of the foot muscles, wearing footwear with poor shock absorption or following the foot or leg being in plaster cast for extended periods. The symptoms may present very similar to a stress fracture of the metatarsals. There may be callous formed on the metatarsal heads. Pain will be reduced if the metatarsal heads are lifted with gentle palpation.

Signs and Symptoms of Metatarsalgia

• Pain present on the sole of the foot in the metatarsal region
• Metatarsal heads may be dropped from their normal position
• Pain will increase with weight bearing
• Callous may form on the metatarsal heads

Treatment of Metatarsalgia

- **RICE** treatment
- Strap the foot with a sponge on the sole to help raise metatarsal heads
- Refer to a neuromuscular therapist / physical therapist
- Refer to hospital if you suspect a stress fracture

Heel Spurs

The heel bone (calcaneus) is the largest bone in the foot, and absorbs the greatest amount of shock and pressure. A heel spur develops as an abnormal growth of the heel bone. Calcium deposits form when the plantar fascia pulls away from the heel area, causing a bony protrusion, or heel spur to develop.

Signs and Symptoms of Heel Spurs

- Pain present under the heel when weight bearing
- Pain will increase with palpation to the area
- A spur (small nodule) may be felt on palpation of the heel

Treatment of Heel Spurs

- RICE treatment
- Strap the foot with a sponge on the sole to cushion the heel
- Refer to a neuromuscular therapist / physical therapist

Athlete's Foot

Athlete's foot is a fungal infection that causes red, dry, flaking skin, sometimes accompanied by pain or itching. The condition usually occurs between the toes or on the soles or sides of the feet. The infection is often contracted in showers, gyms, dressing rooms, swimming pool lockers, or other warm, damp areas where fungus can thrive.

Signs and Symptoms of Athlete's Foot

- Redness
- Dry flaking skin
- Soreness
- Pain
- Itching of the area

Prevention of Athlete's Foot

- Vigilant foot hygiene
- Regular washing of the feet with soap and water and thorough drying, especially between the toes
- Wear clean, dry, airy shoes and socks; never borrow
- Use of medicated foot powders
- Wear protective foot covers while in showers and pools

Treatment of Athlete's Foot

- Dress the foot with a sterile dressing and bandage
- Refer to a doctor

Anterior Compartment Pain

This condition is caused by overuse of the muscles of the forefoot. The muscle sheath becomes tight and inflamed.

Signs and Symptoms of Anterior Compartment Pain

- Pain in anterior and lateral muscles of the lower leg
- Pain increasing with long periods of exercise
- Tender to touch at the site of the inflammation

Treatment of Anterior Compartment Pain

- **RICE** treatment
- Refer to a neuromuscular therapist

Posterior Compartment Pain

This condition is caused by overuse of the calf muscles. The muscle sheath becomes tight and inflamed.

Signs and Symptoms of Posterior Compartment Pain

- Pain in posterior muscles of the lower leg
- Pain increasing with long periods of exercise
- Tender to touch at the site of the inflammation

Treatment of Posterior Compartment Pain

- **RICE** treatment
- Refer to a neuromuscular therapist / physical therapist

Shin Splints

This condition is caused by overuse and tearing of the muscles of the tibial attachment. The muscle attachment site becomes tight and inflamed.

Signs and Symptoms of Shin Splints

- Pain at medial or lateral side of the tibia, or between the tibia and fibula
- Pain increasing with exercise and reducing with rest
- Tender to touch at the site of the inflammation along the bone
- May be accompanied by a stress fracture

Treatment of Shin Splints

- **RICE** treatment
- Referral to a neuromuscular therapist / physical therapist
- Slow build up of exercise programme by therapist

Achilles Tendon Strain

The Achilles tendon is subjected to a number of overuse conditions. Repetitive overloading of tendinous structures leads to inflammation that overwhelms the tissues ability to repair itself. Factors such as faulty biomechanics, poor cushioning of shoes, or excessive downhill running, all contribute to inflammation.

Signs and Symptoms of Achilles Tendon Strain

- Sharp pain at tendon site (posterior ankle area)
- Pain increasing when attempting to rise on to tip toe
- Tender to touch at site
- May be accompanied by a stress fracture

Treatment of Achilles Tendon Strain

- **RICE** treatment
- Refer to a neuromuscular therapist / physical therapist

Tennis Elbow (Lateral Epicondylitis)

This is a condition when the outer part of the elbow becomes painful and tender, usually as a result of a specific strain, overuse, or a direct bang. Sometimes no specific cause is found.

Signs and Symptoms of Tennis Elbow

- Pain at the lateral region of the elbow
- Tender to touch
- May swell
- Movements of the elbow will increase pain
- Lifting will increase pain

Treatment of Tennis Elbow

• **RICE** treatment
• Refer to a neuromuscular therapist / physical therapist

Golfer's Elbow (Medial Epicondylitis)

This is a condition when the inner part of the elbow becomes painful and tender, usually as a result of a specific strain, overuse, or a direct bang. Sometimes no specific cause is found.

Signs and Symptoms of Golfer's Elbow

• Pain at the medial region of the elbow
• Tender to touch
• May swell
• Movements of the elbow will increase pain
• Lifting will increase pain

Treatment of Golfer's Elbow

• **RICE** treatment
• Refer to a neuromuscular therapist / physical therapist

Carpal Tunnel Syndrome

Carpal tunnel syndrome is a condition where compression of the median nerve, as it passes through the wrist into the hand, leads to pain, and tingling in the hand. Sporting activities that predispose athletes to this condition include those that involve repetitive or continuous flexion and extension of the wrist, such as cycling, throwing and racket sports, archery, and gymnastics.

Signs and Symptoms of Carpal Tunnel Syndrome

• Pain in the hand
• Numbness
• Pins and needles in the hand, affecting the thumb, forefinger, middle finger and the upper half of the ring finger
• Weakness in some movements of the thumb
• Pain may extend up into the lower end of the forearm

Treatment of Carpal Tunnel Syndrome

• **RICE** treatment
• Refer to a neuromuscular therapist / physical therapist

Prevention Tips

Reducing the risk of exercise-related injuries is easy if you learn how to exercise correctly. For most people, they believe in a "no pain, no gain" philosophy. If their bodies are not sore the next day, then they did not work out hard enough or long enough. It is vital when exercising or taking part in sporting activities, that we take heed of coaches, therapists and fitness instructors. Warming up and cooling down correctly will dramatically reduce the risk of being injured during play. It is worth preparing correctly for the extra few minutes that it takes to do these exercises compared to months of pain and therapy during injury.

Follow the Safe Sport philosophy, "Look after yourself, exercise correctly, wear protective equipment when necessary and most important, enjoy your time in sport." Here are some tips to help you. For further information, consult your therapist / fitness instructor.

Prevention of Knee Injuries

• Wear correct shoes with soft, flexible soles that fit correctly
• Bend your knees when landing from a jump
• Avoid locking your knees during exercise and play
• Do not bend knees past 90 degrees when doing half knee bends or squats
• Avoid twisting knees by keeping the feet flat as much as possible, especially during exercise and warm ups
• Always use a soft surface when you exercise

Prevention of Muscle Soreness

Muscle soreness is a symptom of having worked out too hard or too long:

- Always warm up correctly and follow the advise of coaches and fitness instructors
- The "no pain, no gain" philosophy is untrue and should not be used
- As well as warming up muscles, it is important to cool them down correctly

Prevention of Blisters

- Get your foot fitted with the correct size footwear
- Wear good sports socks that fit well
- Bathe your feet regularly
- Wear preventive taping, if necessary

Prevention of Side Stitch

Side stitch is a sharp pain felt underneath the ribcage.

- Never eat or drink within 3–4 hours prior to activity
- Breathe correctly during exercise
- If you experience pain during activity, STOP immediately. Never work through it

Prevention of Shin Splints

Shin splints are mild-to-severe aches in front of the lower leg.

- Warm up all leg muscles correctly
- Vary leg exercises to build muscles and minimise overuse of individual muscles

Prevention of Achilles Tendon Pain

Achilles tendon pain is caused by a stretch, tear, or irritation to the tendon that connects the calf muscles to the back of the heel.

- Warm up the tendon correctly
- Shock absorption shoes should be worn
- Get your foot fitted with correct footwear
- Always use a soft surface when you exercise
- Run on flat surfaces instead of uneven ground. Running on uneven ground aggravates the stress put on the Achilles tendon

There are many other similar soft tissue injuries that affect athletes on a regular basis, but it is vital when treating these injuries that if you have any concern that there is an under-lying fracture present, treat it as so, and refer to hospital.

When referring a patient to a neuromuscular therapist, it is important to treat the patient with **RICE** following an injury and arrange the appointment approximately 72 hours after the injury. This allows the **RICE** treatment to reduce swelling and inflammation allowing the therapist to commence treatment sooner.

It is important to understand that the principle of the **RICE** treatment is a guideline for general injury management. However, it is important to understand that when you see the term **ICE**, it is generally a cold compress that we are referring to. Such a cold compress may be made up of gauze, or fabric soaked in chilled water (known as cold therapy), minimising the risk of ice burns to the athlete. As a Sports First Aid Practitioner you should contact your local neuromuscular therapist / physical therapist and discuss a referral system with them.

8. Spinal Injuries

Sports and Your Spine

Exercise is essential to a healthy lifestyle, and for many people sport is the most obvious choice for them to achieve this goal. For people with back injuries, they should consult their doctor before taking up, or returning to sport regardless of how minor the injury. For athletes playing any sport it is important for them to be aware of the strain sport can have on their back and spine. Up to 20% of all injuries that occur in sports involve the lower back or neck. The areas of the spine most at risk are the cervical and lumbar spine. It is most common for the cervical spine to be damaged in contact sports, e.g. rugby or judo and the lumbar spine may be injured in sports that place great stress on that region, e.g. weight-lifting. However, any part of the spine may be damaged once sufficient force is applied. For every sport, a thorough warm up should be completed before starting to play. The warm up should be specific to the muscles used in that sport, but it should also prepare the back and neck for the stresses they may encounter.

The vertebral column consists of 33 vertebrae and the spinal cord runs along the inside of this column. A fracture to any of these bones could lead to the spinal cord being torn or snapped. IT IS VITAL NOT TO MOVE A PATIENT WHEN TREATING THEM WITH A SPINAL INJURY OR SUSPECTED SPINAL INJURY UNLESS THEIR LIFE IS IN DANGER, e.g. fire, gas in the air, lying in the prone position and breathing becoming inhibited.

The major injury types are:

Hyperextension:	The head is wrenched back relative to the body
Hyperflexion:	The head is wrenched forward relative to the body
Lateral flexion:	The head is wrenched to one side relative to the body
Compression:	Impact from above, squashing the casualty's head onto their body
Penetrating:	Injury such as a knife wound which penetrates the spinal column and transacts the spinal cord
Distraction:	"Pulling the head off" injury where the neck is wrenched into traction

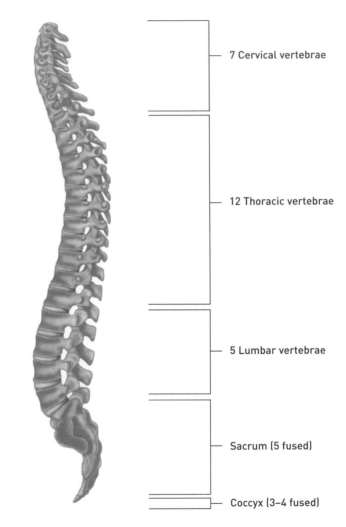

7 Cervical vertebrae

12 Thoracic vertebrae

5 Lumbar vertebrae

Sacrum (5 fused)

Coccyx (3–4 fused)

Figure 8.1: The vertebral column (spine, lateral view).

Signs and Symptoms of Spinal Injuries

• History of the accident (which way did they fall); (how high were they); (which way did they receive the impact)

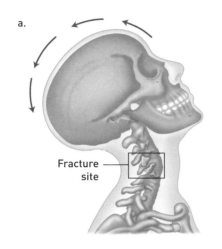

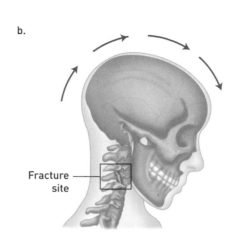

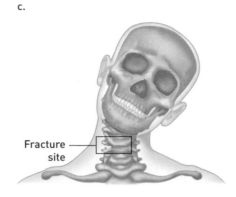

Figure 8.2: The different types of spinal injury; a) hyperextension, b) hyperflexion, c) lateral flexion, d) compression, e) penetrating, f) distraction.

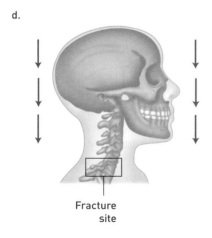

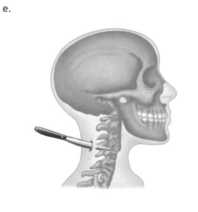

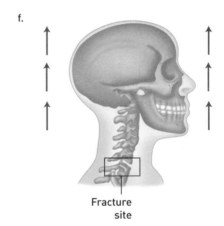

- Patient may feel dull or severe pain in the neck or back
- Swelling at the site of the injury (examine anterior, posterior and lateral aspects of the neck to find swelling, as it will vary depending on the way the neck has broken)
- Deformity at fracture site
- Acute spasms of the back muscles resulting in the area becoming rigid
- Patient may feel a sense of being cut in half

- Tenderness in muscles
- Patient may lose sensation inferiorly to the break site (from neck, chest, waist downwards)
- May lose control of bodily functions
- Patient may become unconscious due to trauma in the body
- Shock

Principle Treatment and Bandaging of Spinal Injuries

• Immobilize the head and neck. (The head lock should not move from this position until medical assistance arrives and takes over or they may ask you to remain locked on while they apply a neck collar and transfer the patient to a spinal board)
• Monitor A, B, C's

If there are 2 Sports First Aid Practitioners:

• Carefully apply a broad-fold bandage around the knees
• Carefully apply a figure of 8 bandage around the ankles
• Carefully immobilise arms to the body
• Treat shock
• Call for an ambulance

If the patient is in the prone position and breathing becomes inhibited due to injury or compression of the lungs, the patient must be log rolled to the supine position (THIS SHOULD NOT BE ATTEMPTED ON YOUR OWN). This procedure requires at least 4 people. As a Sports First Aid Practitioner you should teach and practice this movement with various members of the club in case of emergency. You can use them to assist.

Head and Neck Stabilisation

• Diagnose the injuries
• Treat any bleeding to the body
• Call for an ambulance
• Lie down on your stomach and extend your arms out
• Place your hands either side of the head
• Place your thumb superior to the ear and the rest of your hand inferior to the ear
• Apply gentle medial pressure to the head (press both hands at the same time to minimise movement)
• If airway becomes inhibited, perform a jaw thrust to maintain the airway

• Stay in this position until medical professionals take over the scene and tell you to release. Follow their instructions carefully

The Log Roll

Step 1

With the Sports First Aid Practitioner on the head stabilisation, Sports First Aid Practitioner 2 should kneel at the patient's mid torso and gently straighten the patient's arms with their palms facing inwards towards their body. (Facing the palms outwards may lead to elbow joint damage during the log roll). No. 2 then grasps the patient on the opposite side at the shoulder and just superior to the elbow joint. No. 3 kneels next to No. 2 and grasps the patient at the pelvis and the ankles (by securing a figure of 8 triangular bandage to secure the ankles). No. 4 kneels on the opposite side of the patient at pelvis level and grasps the upper arm (mid third) and the upper leg (mid third).

Step 2

No. 1 at the head is in charge and no member of the team should move unless directed by him. On his command, the patient is rolled onto their side (90 degrees from the ground). This should be done slowly and steadily so that No. 1 can rotate exactly at the same time as the torso. At this stage, the shirt may be cut away to examine the back and a blanket should be laid flat on the ground before the patient is fully lowered (this will help keep the patient warm and assist with the treatment of shock). No. 1 then calls to finish the move and the patient is lowered onto the floor, whilst No. 1 maintains the lock on the head. No. 1 must remain in this position until medical professionals arrive and take command of the scene. Follow their instructions and do not release until they tell you to do so, as they will need to put on an extrication collar and use other spinal equipment.

9. Head Injuries

The Brain

The brain is composed of soft, delicate structures that lie within the rigid skull. Surrounding the brain is a tough, leathery outer covering called the *duramater* (*Latin*: hard mother). Within the brain are (cranial) nerves that are responsible for many activities, such as eye opening, facial movements, speech and hearing. These nerves carry and receive messages that allow the person to think and function normally. There are also centres that control levels of consciousness and vital activities, such as breathing. Blood and spinal fluid inside the skull cavity cushion the brain. When the skull receives a sudden impact, the brain is bounced around the skull cavity and banged against the bones of the skull, causing damage to this system and normal activity of the brain is disturbed.

A brain injury can occur when the skull is struck with enough force to cause the brain to bounce around inside the skull. When the skull is struck, the brain will begin to swell inside the skull with little space to expand. This increased pressure inside the skull results in changes that interfere with the functioning of the brain. If you suspect brain injury in an individual, seek urgent medical attention. The victim needs to be transported to hospital for immediate treatment. Following impact to the head, vision problems, bleeding from the eyes or ears also require urgent medical attention.

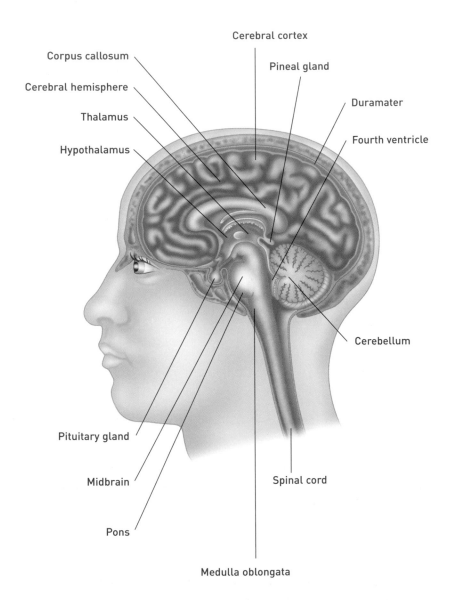

Figure 9.1: The brain and duramater.

Unconsciousness

Unconsciousness is a state of unawareness (loss of consciousness) in which the person is unable to respond to people and other stimuli around them. Often, this is called a *coma / comatose state.*

Altered mental status may accompany early levels of unconsciousness; this would be known as a *state of stupor.* Such changes include sudden confusion, disorientation, dizziness, feeling of nausea and may feel faint.

Unconsciousness and any other SUDDEN change in mental status must be treated as a medical emergency; it is vital that the patient is examined by a doctor to determine the cause of this state. Urgent removal to hospital should be arranged.

If someone is awake but less alert than usual, an easy way to test for change in mental status is to ask a few simple questions:

- What is your name?
- Where do you live?
- What is the date?
- How old are you?

If the person doesn't know or answers incorrectly, then his mental status is diminished. This questioning would be known as *verbal stimuli.*

On examination of the patient, if there is an injury that they should feel pain, but do not, then this shows that their pain stimuli is diminished. The primary cause of this condition is a reduced supply of oxygen to the brain.

Causes of Unconsciousness

- Blow to the head
- Convulsions due to raised temperature (in young children)
- Asphyxia – lack of oxygen to the tissues of the body
- Head injuries – concussion, compression

- Shock – lack of oxygen to the brain
- Stroke – damage to the brain caused by ruptured blood vessels
- Heart attack – damage to muscles of the heart

Signs and Symptoms of Unconsciousness

Patient will be unresponsive to:

- Pain stimulation
- Verbal stimulation

Shock will be present.

Treatment of Unconsciousness

- Call for an ambulance
- Check C spine for injuries
- Open the airway
- Check the breathing and pulse (if not present, call for a cardiac ambulance). Commence BLS protocols
- Commence primary survey
- Diagnose and treat any bleeding
- Commence secondary survey
- Diagnose and treat any fractures
- Place the patient in the recovery position
- Monitor and record vital signs
- Treat for shock

Concussion

Concussion occurs when the brain is shaken inside the skull causing a disturbance to its normal activity. This can be caused by direct or indirect force to the head.

Signs and Symptoms of Concussion

- Patient may lose consciousness briefly
- Memory loss for the time leading up to the accident
- Patient may feel nauseous or vomit
- Patient may feel dizzy and experience some blurred vision
- Patient may have a headache
- Shock

Stages of Concussion

Stage 1: Mild concussion occurs when the person does not lose consciousness, but may seem dazed.

Stage 2: The slightly more severe form of concussion occurs when the person does not lose consciousness but has a period of confusion and does not recall the event.

Stage 3: The classic concussion, which is the most severe form, occurs when the person loses consciousness for a brief period of time and has no memory of the event.

Treatment of Concussion

- Check C spine for injuries
- Open the airway
- Check the breathing and pulse (if not present, call for a cardiac ambulance). Commence BLS protocols
- Commence primary survey
- Diagnose and treat any bleeding
- Commence secondary survey
- Diagnose and treat any fractures
- Place the patient in the recovery position
- Monitor and record vital signs
- Treat for shock
- Call for an ambulance

Compression

Compression occurs when pressure is applied internally or externally to the brain. Internal pressure may be caused by bleeding in the brain or swelling of the brain. External pressure may be caused by a depressed (complicated) fracture of the skull or a heavy object lying on the skull. The main concern in a head injury is that there may be bleeding inside the skull. This can occur even if the skull is not clearly damaged. The accumulation of blood may eventually put pressure on the brain and cause brain damage. Head injuries are often not serious, but brain injuries can be.

Signs and Symptoms of Compression

- Patient will gradually lose consciousness
- Patient will have slow, noisy breathing
- Patient will have a slow, full pulse
- Eyes will be unequal and unresponsive (one eye may be pin-pointed)
- Memory loss for the time leading up to the accident
- Patient may vomit
- Patient may feel dizzy and may experience some blurred vision
- Patient may have a headache
- Bleeding may become present from the ears mixed with a straw-coloured fluid (CSF, cerebrospinal fluid)
- Bleeding may become visible from the nose
- Shock

Treatment of Compression

- Check C spine for injuries
- Open the airway
- Check the breathing and pulse (if not present, call for a cardiac ambulance). Commence BLS protocols
- Diagnose and treat any fractures
- Diagnose and treat any wounds

- Maintain an open airway
- Apply pads to facilitate fluid loss from ears (do not stop this flow)
- Treat for shock
- Place the patient in the recovery position on the injured side
- Monitor and record vital signs
- Call for an ambulance

Any athlete who you suspect has a head injury, should be removed from play at once and examined by a medical doctor.

10. Chest Injuries

The Ribcage

Ribs are composed of successive layers of flat bone, which give the ribs their flexibility or 'spring'. The ribcage protects many of our vital organs like the heart and lungs. Each of us has 12 pairs. The pairs are broken up into 2 sections, called the *true* and *false* ribs. True ribs are located superior in the ribcage and are the first 7 pairs, which attach anteriorly to the sternum. The inferior ribs, known as the false ribs consist of the inferior 5 pairs. Pairs 8, 9 and 10 are attached anteriorly with cartilage to pair 7 at the inferior aspect of the sternum, and the remaining 2 pairs known as *floating* ribs do not attach anteriorly to the sternum. All 12 pairs attach posteriorly to the spinal column. When ribs fracture, often the 'spring' is reduced, rather than the entire bone being detached from the spinal column or the sternum. Rib injuries cause distress due to the difficulty the patient has in breathing. All rib injuries should be treated as life-threatening and checked by a doctor immediately.

Fractured Ribs

A closed fracture to the rib occurs normally by direct force.

Signs and Symptoms of Fractured Ribs

- History of force to the chest
- Pale, cool skin
- Pain at the site, especially when breathing in
- Rapid pulse
- Rapid shallow breathing
- 'Guarding' of the injury

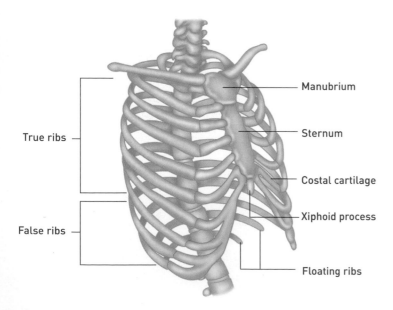

Figure 10.1: The ribcage.

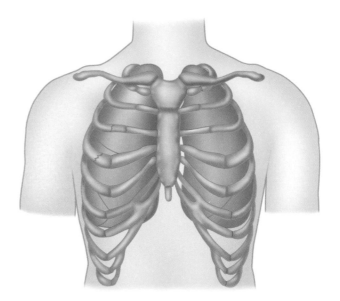

Figure 10.2: Fractured ribs.

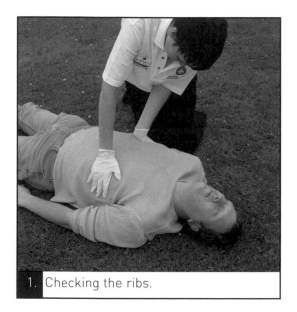

1. Checking the ribs.

Treatment of Fractured Ribs

- A, B, C's
- Examine the ribs (*see* photograph 1)
- Apply ice to the injured site
- Put the arm on the injured side in an elevation sling to act as a splint
- Place a broad fold bandage around the elbow and tie around the torso
- Refer to hospital
- Treat for shock
- Monitor vital signs

Flail Chest

A flail chest occurs when a segment of the thoracic wall becomes unattached from the rest of the chest wall. This most typically occurs when ribs are fractured in two places, allowing that segment of the thoracic wall to "float" independently of the rest of the chest wall. Chest wall motion best describes a flail chest.

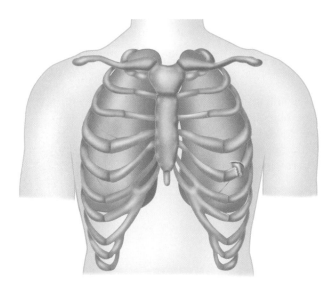

Figure 10.3: Complicated rib fracture.

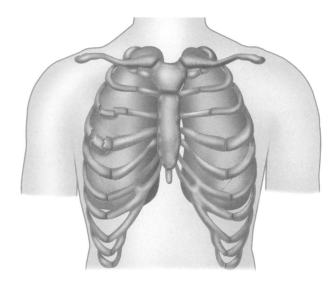

Figure 10.4: Flail chest.

Signs and Symptoms of Flail Chest

- Pale, cool, clammy skin
- Rapid, weak pulse
- Shallow, difficult breathing
- Paradoxical chest movements, where the injured area moves in the opposite direction to the rest of the chest
- Cyanosis
- Pain, especially when breathing in
- Visible hollow area

Treatment of Flail Chest

- A, B, C's
- Apply a firm pad over the flail section ideally using a small SAM® Splint
- Apply a firm bandage in place. (Do not tie it too tight and restrict breathing)
- Incline the patient to the injured side
- Call for an ambulance

Penetrating Chest Wound

A penetrating chest wound may be a wound where the object is still in place in the wall of the chest, or it may be an open wound left by the object, e.g. a stab wound. If the object is still in place, DO NOT remove it. Follow the guideline for open fracture treatments. If it is too long or too awkward to manage, call the fire service to have it cut, but never attempt to remove or cut the object yourself.

Signs and Symptoms of a Penetrating Chest Wound

- History of the accident
- Object still in place
- Open wound in the chest wall (look for both entry and exit wounds) bleeding from this wound may be filled with air bubbles as air is sucked in through the hole in the chest wall
- Blood may appear in the mouth if the lung is punctured
- Pale, cool, clammy skin
- Rapid, weak pulse
- Rapid, shallow breathing
- Cyanosis
- Pain at the site

Treatment of a Penetrating Chest Wound

- A, B, C's
- If the object is still in place, stabilise with a pad around the entry wound
- If an open wound, apply plastic or a non-stick pad, taped on three sides, only leaving the bottom side untaped to allow for air to escape from the chest
- If conscious, incline the patient towards the injured side with blankets to support them
- If unconscious, place the patient in the recovery position on the injured side
- Call for an ambulance
- Treat for shock
- Monitor vital signs

11. Medical Emergencies

Fainting

Fainting is a brief loss of consciousness due to a reduced blood supply to the brain. Episodes may last from a couple of seconds or up to an hour. Any episode that lasts for more than a few minutes should be checked by a doctor. A doctor should also check a person experiencing regular episodes.

Causes of Fainting

• Low blood sugar (hypoglycaemia)
• Any condition in which there is a rapid loss of blood. This can be from internal or external bleeding
• Toxic shock syndrome
• Heart and circulatory problems such as abnormal heart rhythm, heart attacks, high or low blood pressure or stroke
• Heat stroke or heat exhaustion
• Eating disorders such as anorexia, bulimia
• A sudden change in body position like standing up too quickly (postural hypotension)
• Extreme pain following injury or during illness
• Sudden emotional shock
• Long periods of time in hot and humid weather

Signs and Symptoms of Fainting

• Dizziness
• Temporary loss of consciousness
• May feel nauseous
• May see spots in front of the eyes
• Feeling of weakness
• Temporary disorientation
• Shock

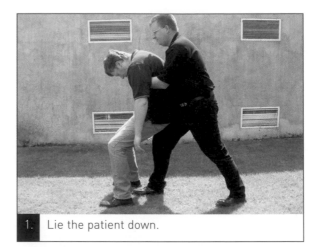

1. Lie the patient down.

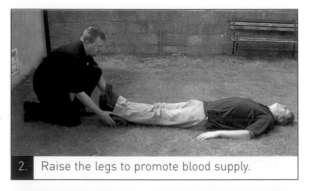

2. Raise the legs to promote blood supply.

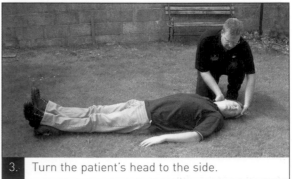

3. Turn the patient's head to the side.

Treatment of Fainting

- Lie the patient down (*see* photograph 1)
- Raise the legs to promote blood supply to the brain (*see* photograph 2)
- Turn the victim's head to the side, so that the tongue doesn't fall back into the throat and to facilitate the drainage of vomit (*see* photograph 3)
- Loosen any tight clothing (neck, chest and waist)
- Sponge the person's face and neck with cool water
- Treat shock

Do not allow the patient to stand up suddenly. Never give fluids to a person until they are fully conscious.

Sunburn

Sunburn occurs due to burning of the first layer of the skin. It is caused when the skin is exposed to too much sunlight. Burn times vary according to skin types. You should always protect yourself with a sun block or sun protective cream. Sunburn is painful, so cover up.

Signs and Symptoms of Sunburn

- Reddening of the skin
- Blisters may appear depending on the level of the burn
- Pain
- Tender to touch
- Headache
- Fatigue
- Nausea
- Swelling

Treatment of Sunburn

- Take a cool bath or shower
- Apply an aloe vera lotion several times a day

- Leave blisters intact to speed healing and avoid infection. If they burst, apply an antibacterial cream on the open areas. Cover with a sterile gauze dressing
- Avoid any exposure to sunlight
- If the person feels nauseous or begins vomiting, dizzy or any other complications appear, visit the GP for examination

Heat Exhaustion

Sweat acts as our natural air conditioning system. As sweat evaporates from our skin, it cools our body temperature. Our personal cooling system can fail during excessive exercise. When this happens, our body heat can climb to dangerous levels. This can result in heat exhaustion or a heat stroke, which is life threatening.

Heat exhaustion takes time to develop. Fluids and salt are vital for our health. It is very important to drink lots of liquids before, during and after exercise. You should consult your medical practitioner for advice.

Signs and Symptoms of Heat Exhaustion

- Cool, clammy, pale skin
- Sweating
- Dry mouth
- Fatigue, weakness
- Dizziness
- Headache
- Nausea, sometimes vomiting
- Muscle cramps
- Weak and rapid pulse

Treatment of Heat Exhaustion

- Treat shock
- Monitor vital signs

- Give sips of water to the patient
- Arrange for a medical practitioner to assess the patient

Heat Stroke

Heat stroke, unlike heat exhaustion, strikes suddenly, with little warning. When the body's cooling system fails, the body's temperature rises fast. This creates an emergency condition.

Signs and Symptoms of Heat Stroke

- Very high temperature
- Hot, dry, red skin
- No sweating
- Deep breathing and fast pulse, then shallow breathing and weak pulse
- Dilated pupils
- Confusion, delirium, hallucinations
- Convulsions
- Loss of consciousness

Treatment of Heat Stroke

- Treat shock
- Monitor vital signs
- Sponge the patient with tepid water
- Call for an ambulance

Tips for the Prevention of Heat Exhaustion and Heat Stroke

- Take caution when you exercise or play in the sun. At the first sign of heat exhaustion, get out of the sun otherwise your body temperature will continue to rise
- Do not exercise vigorously on very hot days
- Wear light, loose fitting clothing, such as cotton, so that sweat can evaporate. This process should never be restricted

- Drink lots of liquids, especially if your urine is a dark yellow colour, to replace the fluids you lose from sweating
- Drink water or a recommended sports drink (especially if you sweat a lot)
- Do not drink alcohol, beverages or caffeine for 24 hours before an event, because they speed up fluid loss
- Thirst is not a reliable sign that your body needs fluids. When you exercise, it is better to sip rather than gulp the liquids
- Know the signs of heat stroke and heat exhaustion and don't ignore them

Poisoning

A poison is any substance that enters the body and causes harm to the body.

Types of Poisoning

Corrosive: Any substance that will burn the patient once taken, such as chemicals, bleach or acid

Non-corrosive: Any substance that enters the body that does not cause burning, such as drugs, smoke, or tablets

How the Poisons Enter the Body?

Poisons can enter the body in a number of ways, either accidentally or intentionally:

Ingestion: Through the mouth by eating or drinking poisonous substances

Inhalation: Through the lungs by inhaling household or industrial gases, chemical vapours, or fumes from fires, stoves and exhaust pipes

Injection: By injection into the skin as the result of bites from some animals, insects, poisonous fish, or by hypodermic syringe

Absorption: Through the skin after contact with poisonous sprays such as pesticides, insecticides, chemicals, or creams

Splash in the eye: Any substance that comes into contact with the eye such as chemical sprays, or poisonous liquid substances

Treatment of Poisoning

- If the patient is conscious, quickly ask them what has happened
- Try to assess what drugs or substances they have taken (look for bottles of tablets, needles, etc.)
- Do not attempt to induce vomiting. If the lips or mouth show signs of burning, cool them by giving the patient water or milk to drink. Burning of the lips and mouth will suggest that a corrosive poison has been consumed
- If the patient has taken non-corrosive poison, induce vomiting
- Once a patient has vomited, collect a sample and take it to the hospital so that it can be examined to determine the drug(s) / poison(s) that have been taken
- If the patient is unconscious, but breathing normally, place in the recovery position
- If the breathing and heartbeat stop, begin resuscitation immediately

N.B. Take care not to contaminate yourself with any poison that may be around the casualty's mouth. USE YOUR SHIELD
- Call for an ambulance
- Send to the hospital with the patient any samples of vomit and containers such as bottles or pillboxes found nearby

Drug Poisoning

This condition is caused by accidental overdose or drug abuse.

Signs and Symptoms of Drug Poisoning

- History of drugs being taken
- These will vary according to the drug and the quantity taken

- Vomit will be expected
- The pupils of the eyes may be abnormally dilated or contracted
- The level of consciousness will be impaired
- The patient may become unconscious
- The heart may stop beating

Treatment of Drug Poisoning

- Follow the general treatment for poisoning
- Check arms for needle marks; look for empty tablet bottles
- Call for an ambulance
- Be prepared to resuscitate
- Take the poison container to hospital

Snake Bites (see photograph 4)

Snake bites are uncommon in the UK and Ireland but should be treated with extreme care if encountered. Following the bite, the symptoms of poisoning may take several hours to develop depending on the breed of snake.

Signs and Symptoms of Snake Bites

- History of snake bite
- A noticeable bite on the skin, or may appear as nothing more than a discoloration
- Pain and swelling in the area of the bite
- Rapid pulse and laboured breathing
- Progressive general weakness
- Vision problems (dim or blurred)
- Nausea and vomiting
- Convulsions
- Drowsiness or unconsciousness
- Breathing and pulse may stop

Treatment of Snake Bites

- Keep the patient calm
- Treat for shock, maintain body heat
- Call for an ambulance and contact the poison control centre
- Locate the fang marks and clean the site with antiseptic and water
- Remove any jewellery from the bitten limb
- Place the patient in a half sitting position to raise them above the bite area
- Keep any bitten extremities immobilised. The application of a splint will help to keep the bite at the level of the heart, or when this is not possible, below the level of the heart
- Apply a light-constricting band above and below the wound. This is to restrict the flow of lymph, not the flow of blood (*see* photograph 5)

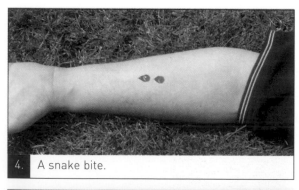

4. A snake bite.

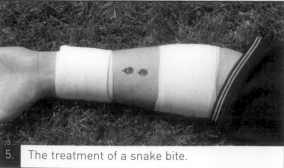

5. The treatment of a snake bite.

- Monitor vital signs
- NEVER ATTEMPT TO SUCK OUT POISON. YOU WILL POISON YOURSELF

Asthma

Asthma is a chronic, inflammatory disease in which the airways become sensitive to allergens (any substance that triggers an allergic reaction). People with asthma have extra-sensitive airways. Triggers like dust, pollens, animals, tobacco smoke and exercise may make their airways swell and narrow, causing wheezing, coughing and difficulty breathing. This is known as an *asthma attack*.

Signs and Symptoms of Asthma

- History of asthma
- The lining of the airways become swollen and inflamed
- The muscles that surround the airways tighten
- Diagnosed sufferer
- Coughing
- Wheezing
- Shortness of breath
- Gasping for air
- Shock

Treatment of Asthma

- Encourage and assist the patient to take their inhaler
- Maintain an open airway
- Monitor vital signs
- Treat shock
- If the attack is severe and the airways become obstructed, call for an ambulance
- Be prepared to resuscitate

Diabetes

The *pancreas* is a small digestive organ that, in addition to other functions, manufactures *insulin*, a chemical necessary for normal functioning of the cells in the body. Diabetes is a condition where the pancreas does not produce: a sufficient amount of insulin at the right time; an incorrect amount of insulin; or, any insulin, resulting in an imbalance of blood sugar levels in the body. If insulin is not present in the blood, any sugar (glucose) that has been produced by the digestion and processing of food cannot be transmitted into cells. This results in excessive glucose in the blood, while the cells have insufficient food for normal function. This is corrected by diet and by the regular taking of small doses of insulin or, in mild diabetes, by medication which stimulates the action of the pancreas. Type 1 diabetes generally develops in people under twenty and carries the risk of long-term damage to the eyes and circulation. Type 2 diabetes generally develops after the age of 40, and is much more common.

Signs and Symptoms of Diabetes

- Dizzy or light headedness
- Pale and / or sweaty skin
- The patient may become unconscious
- Confusion
- Agitation
- Irregular breathing patterns
- Thirst
- Frequent urination
- May have a sweet smell from the breath
- Drowsiness – if the patient is alert, ask how you can help them
- Call for an ambulance
- Do not give insulin. If the patient is conscious, you may assist them to inject themselves

Types of Diabetes

Hyperglycaemia: This is a result of excess glucose in the blood – high blood sugar. This may occur with un-treated diabetes or diabetics not regulating their diet or medication. If untreated, this condition will worsen and result in unconsciousness or death.

Hypoglycaemia: This is a result of decreased glucose in the blood – low blood sugar and may worsen rapidly. If untreated, hypoglycaemia may, in a short time, result in loss of consciousness or death.

Treatment of Diabetes

If the patient is conscious:

- Assist them to check their blood sugar levels
- If blood sugar levels are low, give them a sugary drink
- Assist them to take their medication
- Reassure them
- Monitor vital signs
- Sit them in a half seated position (*see* photograph 6)
- Treat shock

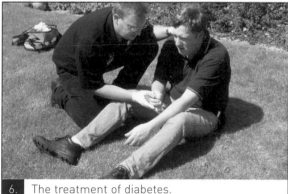

6. The treatment of diabetes.

If the patient is unconscious:

• Maintain an open airway
• Place in the recovery position
• Monitor vital signs
• Treat for shock
• Be prepared to resuscitate
• Call for an ambulance

NEVER GIVE INSULIN TO A PATIENT.
THIS SHOULD ONLY BE DONE BY A DOCTOR

Epilepsy

Epilepsy is a brain disorder involving recurrent seizures. The seizures are caused by abnormal electrical activity in the brain. Epilepsy can affect people of any age. Most seizures happen without warning, last only a short time and stop without any special treatment. Injuries can occur, but most people do not come to any harm in a seizure and do not usually need to go to hospital or see a doctor.

When a person has a convulsive seizure it is possible that their regular breathing pattern will be affected and they may go blue. Although this can be frightening to witness, it does not usually mean it is a medical emergency.

Risk factors of developing epilepsy:

• Family history
• Injuries to the head
• Injuries to the brain
• Other medical conditions that have an effect on the brain

Risk factors for people with epilepsy:

• Lack of sleep
• Skipping doses of epilepsy medications
• Use of alcohol or other recreational drugs
• Certain prescribed medications
• Pregnancy
• Chronic infections

Types of Seizures

Simple partial seizures

In this type of seizure, there is no loss of consciousness and the person is aware of what is happening to them. However, the seizure's effects can be disturbing for the person experiencing them and reassurance should be given to the patient. If this type of seizure is a warning – sometimes called an *aura* – that a convulsive seizure will follow, the person may require assistance to get into a safe position while the seizure is in progress. To minimise the risk of further injury you should lie them down carefully and remove any objects that may cause them injury.

Complex partial seizures

In a complex partial seizure, the person normally becomes confused, wanders around aimlessly or acts as if they do not understand what they are doing (picks up objects, removes clothes and could cross a road without even looking).

Do not restrain the person, but guide them away from dangerous situations, such as wandering into the road. Speak gently and calmly to help reassure them and reorientation to their surroundings as quickly as possible after the seizure. They may be confused for some time afterwards and it may be better to give the person space rather than to keep offering help that may be misunderstood. Do not crowd them or keep asking them lots of questions, advise them that you are a Sports First Aid Practitioner and are willing to assist them and wait until they are ready to communicate with you.

Absence seizures (previously known as petit mal)

In an absence seizure the person's consciousness is briefly interrupted. This type of seizure is usually very brief. If the person is walking, they may continue and therefore may need to be guided away from danger. Gently and calmly speak to them and reassure them and guide them to safety.

Tonic (stiffening) and atonic (drop) seizures

In these seizures, the person suddenly becomes stiff or their muscles relax. If standing the person falls to the ground and then recovers quickly although they may be confused. Reassure and check for injury. Stay with them until they have fully recovered. If they are badly injured, call for medical assistance.

Treatment of Epilepsy

- Reassure the patient at all times
- Assist them to lie down if a complex seizure is pending
- Guide them to safety if full conscious thought is interrupted
- Do not ask them a lot of questions as they may be confused
- Wait until they are ready to communicate with you (*see* photograph 7)

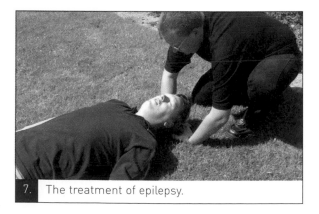

7. The treatment of epilepsy.

In the case of fits:

- Remove any objects that may cause harm to the patient during a fit
- Inter-lock your fingers and glide under the patient's head (do not restrain the head during seizure)
- If a patient loses control of bodily function, cover them with a blanket to protect their privacy and dignity
- Remain in position until the fit stops
- Place the patient in the recovery position
- Call for an ambulance
- Treat for shock
- Monitor vital signs

It is a medical emergency and medical assistance should be sought if:

- The person is injured during the seizure
- Breathing after a seizure remains difficult
- Subsequent seizures occur without breaks
- The seizure continues for longer than is usual for that person
- The seizure is still ongoing after five minutes when it is not known how long they usually last for that person

Anaphylaxis

Anaphylaxis is a rare but severe allergic reaction that occurs suddenly and can be life threatening. Anaphylaxis can happen moments or even seconds after being exposed to a triggering substance. Anaphylaxis, also known as *anaphylactic shock*, is the body's overreaction to a foreign substance. The immune system responds by producing an abundance of antibodies, which are a type of protein created by the white blood cells, to fight the foreign substance. These antibodies, called *immunoglobulin E (IgE)*, cause specific cells to release chemical substances that can be harmful. The release of these chemicals causes allergic symptoms. In the case of anaphylaxis, this can include drastic changes to circulation and air passages similar to those experienced when someone goes into shock. Diagnosed patients will advise that they require medical assistance or assistance to take their medication (epinephrine) as they may have experienced an episode previously.

Signs and Symptoms of Anaphylaxis

- Sense of impending doom
- Hives or rash covering the body
- Tightness of the throat
- Hoarse voice
- Nausea
- Vomiting
- Abdominal pain
- Diarrhoea
- Dizziness or light-headedness
- Cardiac effects, including a rapid drop in blood pressure and irregular heartbeat
- Difficulty breathing
- Swelling of the throat or other body parts
- Unconsciousness
- Heart may stop
- Shock

The symptoms and course of anaphylaxis can vary. Initial signs of an anaphylactic episode can be deceptively mild, such as a runny nose, a skin rash all over the body, a tingling in the throat, or a nondescript "strange feeling". These symptoms can quickly escalate to a major medical emergency situation. It is important to seek immediate emergency medical care if you or someone you know begins to go into anaphylactic shock.

Treatment of Anaphylaxis

- Loosen tight clothing (neck, chest, and waist)
- Place the patient lying down

- Call for an ambulance (advise you suspect an anaphylactic shock)
- If the patient is conscious and has medication, assist them to take it
- If the patient is unconscious, place in the recovery position
- Maintain an open airway
- Be prepared to resuscitate
- Treat shock

Common Trigger Substances of Anaphylaxis

- Medications and drugs
- Food
- Drinks
- Insect bites or stings

Tips for the Prevention of Anaphylaxis

By taking certain foods or medications prior to excess exercise (if you are a diagnosed sufferer of this condition, seek medical advise before taking up exercise) the onset of anaphylaxis should be prevented.

Self-awareness and Treatment of Anaphylaxis

- Call for help
- Lie down in a safe position
- Take your medication
- Know your triggers
- Avoiding the substances to which you are allergic is the most effective way to prevent future anaphylactic episodes
- Know what to do if you unexpectedly come into contact with your trigger
- Your doctor can help you develop a detailed plan of emergency care
- Educate family and friends on what to do if you begin to have an anaphylactic episode
- If your doctor has prescribed a self-inject shot of epinephrine, carry it with you at all times

- Wear a medical bracelet that indicates your anaphylactic triggers
- Never take anything to eat or drink without ensuring that it does not contain your trigger

Frostbite

Frostbite looks like a serious heat burn, but it's actually body tissue that's frozen and, in severe cases, tissue necrosis may occur. Frostbite commonly affects the toes, fingers, earlobes, chin, and tip of the nose. These body parts are often left uncovered and can freeze quickly. Frostbite can happen when temperatures drop below freezing, but wind chill speeds up heat loss and can add to the risk. Both can set in very slowly, or very quickly. This will depend on how long the skin is exposed to the cold and how cold and windy it is.

Signs and Symptoms of Frostbite

- Pain
- Swelling
- White or pale skin
- Numbness
- The skin feels hard and solid
- Blisters may also develop
- Loss of function and absence of pain follow

Treatment of Frostbite

- If the victim is not breathing, do CPR (follow BLS protocols)
- Remove the victim out of the cold and into a warm place
- Remove wet and/or tight clothing
- Remove jewellery
- Warm the affected area by soaking it in a tub of warm water and an antiseptic solution
- Stop when the affected area becomes red, not when sensation returns

- If warm water is not available, cover the victim with blankets etc., or place the affected body part in a warm body area
- Keep exposed area elevated but protected
- Never rub or massage a frostbitten area
- Protect exposed area from the cold. It is more sensitive to re-injury
- Don't burst blisters
- Don't use hot water bottles or electric heating pads

Tips for the Prevention of Frostbite

- Don't drink alcohol or smoke cigarettes
- Wear layers of clothes
- Alcohol causes blood to lose heat quickly
- Smoking slows down blood circulation to the extremities
- Stay indoors as much as possible when it is very cold and windy
- When you are outside, shield your face, etc. from the wind

Frostnip

Frostnip is a less serious problem than frostbite. The skin turns white or pale and feels cold but the skin does not feel hard and solid. Like frostbite, frostnip can happen when temperatures drop below freezing, but wind chill speeds up heat loss and can add to the risk. Both can set in very slowly, or very quickly. This will depend on how long the skin is exposed to the cold and how cold and windy it is.

Treatment of Frostnip

- If the victim is not breathing, do CPR (follow BLS protocols)
- Remove the victim out of the cold and into a warm place
- Remove wet and/or tight clothing
- Remove jewellery
- Warm the affected area by soaking it in a tub of warm water and an antiseptic solution

- Stop when the affected area becomes red, not when sensation returns
- If warm water is not available, cover the victim with blankets etc., or place the affected body part in a warm body area
- Keep exposed area elevated but protected
- Never rub or massage an affected area
- Protect exposed area from the cold. It is more sensitive and may develop to frostbite
- Don't burst blisters
- Don't use hot water bottles or electric heating pads

12. Common Minor Sports Injuries

Black Eyes

Bleeding beneath the skin around the eye causes a black eye (*see* photograph 1). Sometimes a black eye may indicate a more extensive injury, like a skull fracture, compression or brain injury, particularly if the area around both eyes is bruised or if there has been head trauma. You must examine the eyes with a pen light for reaction to the light to check normal responses. If you are ever in doubt, remove the athlete from play and refer to a doctor immediately.

Signs and Symptoms of Black Eyes

- History of impact to the eye or head
- Bruising around the eyelids and surrounding area
- Swelling
- Tender to touch
- Possible blurring of vision
- May feel dizzy
- Eye may close due to swelling

Treatment of Black Eyes

- Apply cold compress (use cold therapy protocols)
- Monitor eye for blood-shot to the eye itself

Seek medical care immediately if vision problems are experienced (double vision, blurring), severe pain, or bleeding in the eye.

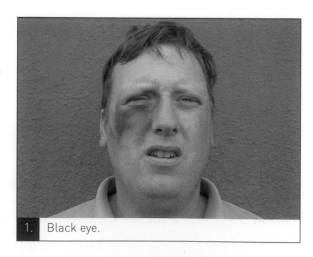

1. Black eye.

Eye Abrasions

The front of the eye is extremely sensitive. Abrasions can be painful (*see* photograph 2).

If the cornea is scratched, it might feel as if there is sand in the eye. It is vital not to rub the eye as this may further scratch the cornea.

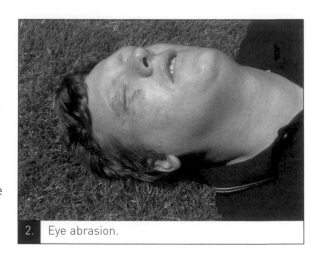

2. Eye abrasion.

Signs and Symptoms of Eye Abrasions

- Tears
- Blurred vision
- Increased sensitivity or redness around the eye
- Pain
- Continuous feeling that there is something in the eye

Treatment of Eye Abrasions

- Apply pads to both eyes. This will stop blinking of the injured eye and minimise further risk to the cornea if grit is still present in the eye
- Refer to hospital

Do not under-estimate eye abrasions, as sight may be damaged if not treated correctly by a doctor.

Nose Bleeds

Nose bleeds are a common condition which usually only result in minor blood loss from blood vessels inside the nostrils (see photograph 3).

More serious bleeding may result in considerable blood loss and, if the patient swallows blood, vomiting may result. With more severe bleeding from the nose, it may indicate head trauma.

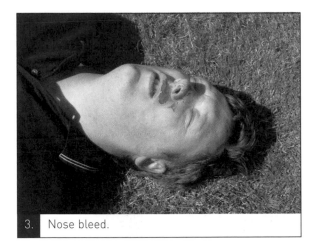

3. Nose bleed.

Signs and Symptoms of Nose Bleeds

- History of impact to the nose
- Bleeding from the nostrils (internal injury)
- Bleeding from the nose itself (external injury)
- Nose bleeds may occur spontaneously or after sneezing, picking or blowing the nose
- If bleeding occurs after an accident, examine for a nose or skull fracture
- Leakage of clear or straw-coloured fluid (CSF) from the nose may indicate a skull fracture

Treatment of Nose Bleeds

- Sit the patient down
- Advise the patient to breathe through the mouth
- Tilt the head forward
- With a sterile dressing, pinch the entire soft part of the nose (this may be done by the patient)
- Until the bleeding has stopped, discourage the patient from talking,

swallowing, coughing, spitting, sniffing or raising the head. Allow any blood to drip into a container held in front of the patient
- Maintain the pressure for a full 10 minutes. If bleeding has not been controlled, consult a doctor
- Have the patient clean around the nose with a swab moistened with warm water
- When the bleeding stops, tell the patient not to blow his nose for at least 4 hours, and to avoid exertion so as to not disturb the clot
- NEVER PLUG AN ATHLETE'S NOSE AND LET THEM RETURN TO PLAY. A doctor should only use nose plugs

Tooth Dislodgement / Broken Teeth

It is common in sporting activities that teeth may be knocked out. While the initial impact will be painful and cause some bleeding the pain normally subsides quickly. In some cases it is possible to have a tooth re-implanted successfully. It is vital to protect the tooth and get to the dentist immediately.

Signs and Symptoms of Tooth Dislodgement / Broken Teeth

- Tooth or part of a tooth broken or dislodged
- Bleeding from the gum
- Pain
- Swelling of the gum
- Possible underlying fracture to the jaw

Treatment of Tooth Dislodgement

- Handle teeth by the top only, not the roots
- Don't rub or scrape the tooth to remove dirt
- Gently rinse the tooth in a bowl of tap water. Don't hold it under running water
- Advise the athlete to replace the tooth in the socket. Then bite down

gently on gauze to help keep it in place

- If the tooth can't be replaced in the socket, place it in a small sterile container. Fill the container with milk, the athlete's own saliva or a warm, mild saltwater solution
- Give the athlete some cotton wool to place in the socket to control bleeding and encourage them to spit out blood from the mouth
- Refer to a dentist or hospital

Treatment of Broken Teeth

- Advise the athlete to spit out the broken pieces
- Place them in a container filled with milk
- Encourage them to spit out any blood from the mouth
- Refer to a dentist or hospital
- If you participate in contact sports, it is advisable to be fitted with mouth shields fitted by your dentist

Ear Injuries

Earache

Earache can be mild or severe. Eustachian tubes go from the back of the throat to the middle ear. When the tube gets blocked, fluid gathers, causing pain. Conditions that make this happen include an infection of the middle ear, colds, sinus infections, and allergies. Other conditions that can cause ear pain include changes in air pressure in a plane, something stuck in the ear, too much earwax, tooth problems, and ear injuries.

Risk Factors of Earache

- A mild ear injury
- Blowing the nose hard or too many times
- Sticking an object of any kind in the ear
- A cold, sinus, or upper respiratory infection

- Swimming, and it is extremely painful when the earlobe is wiggled or touched
- Exposure to extremely loud noises

Signs and Symptoms of Earache

- Pain inside the ear (mild to severe depending on the injury)
- Wax may drain from the ear
- Clear fluid or blood may drain from the ear (possible brain or head injury)
- Any severe ear pain following impact should be referred to hospital

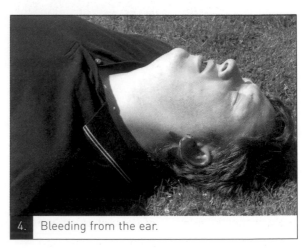

4. Bleeding from the ear.

Treatment of Bleeding from the Ear (*see* photograph 4)

- Place a sterile pad on the ear and secure with a loose bandage (do not stop the flow of blood, fluid or wax)
- Examine the head for injuries (following impact)
- Examine the eyes (following impact)
- Monitor vital signs
- If you suspect a head injury, treat as such and call for an ambulance
- If you suspect minor bleeding, only consult a doctor

Swimmer's Ear

This is an infection of the ear canal, the tubular opening that carries sounds from the outside of the body to the eardrum. Many different types of bacteria or fungi can cause it.

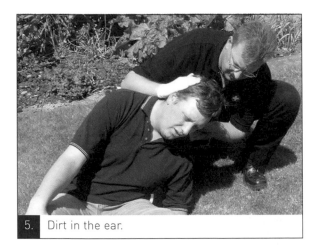
5. Dirt in the ear.

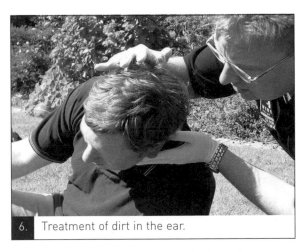
6. Treatment of dirt in the ear.

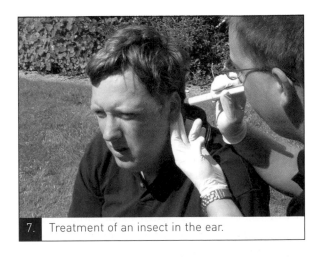
7. Treatment of an insect in the ear.

Prevention and Treatment of Swimmer's Ear

- Wear wax or silicone earplugs that can be softened and shaped to fit the ears
- Wear a swimming cap to help keep water from getting into the ears
- Don't swim in dirty water
- Swim on the surface of the water instead of underneath the water
- Consult a doctor regarding this condition

Treatment of Dirt in the Ear (see photographs 5 & 6)

- Lean the head to the blocked side to allow dirt to fall out
- If the dirt does not come out, consult your doctor

Treatment of an Insect in the Ear (see photograph 7)

- Shining a pen light into the ear may cause the insect to come out
- If the insect does not come out, consult your doctor

Friction Burns

A friction burn occurs when skin is scraped off by contact with a surface such as roads, tarmac or other hard sporting surfaces. It usually is both a scrape (abrasion) and a heat burn. Friction burns are often seen in athletes who fall on floors, courts, or tracks.

Signs and Symptoms of Friction Burns

- History of sliding fall
- Redness of the skin
- Capillary bleeding may be present with an abrasive type wound
- Grit or dirt may be present

Treatment of Friction Burns

- Cleanse the wound with sterile water. Do not try to pick grit out of the wound (this will be done by the hospital as you will cause further damage)
- Apply ice to injured site
- Dress the wound with sterile dressing and bandage

- Never use freeze spray or cool gels if there is a wound present
- Refer to a doctor for tetanus injection

13. Athletes with Disabilities

People-first

Many people with disabilities are heavily involved in sport. As a Sports First Aid Practitioner you should be aware of their needs and be able to respond accordingly. This chapter is dedicated to people with disabilities in the sporting field. I hope that this chapter will raise awareness of the important role people with disabilities play in our society and sporting arenas throughout the world. Athletes with disabilities can be injured just the same as anybody else so here are some important facts about disability for you. If your sporting organisation or club do not have any athletes with disabilities involved why not ask yourselves the following questions:

• Is our club accessible?

• Have we had an access audit carried out on our grounds and facilities?

• Do we have a positive equality action plan in place?

• How can athletes with disabilities access our service?

If you need any assistance with these questions, contact your National Disability Authority for advice and guidance.

People-first language is a language that is both accurate and sensitive. It promotes the use of 'people-first' language – language that puts the focus on the individual, rather than on disability. 'People-first' language helps us remember that people are unique individuals and that their abilities or disabilities are only attributes and do not define who they are.

The following 'people-first' phrases may serve as a helpful guideline:

Affirmative Phrase: person with a disability; people with disabilities
Negative Phrase: the disabled; handicapped; crippled; suffers from a disability

Affirmative Phrase: person who is blind; person with a visual impairment
Negative Phrase: the blind

Affirmative Phrase: person who is deaf; person with a hearing impairment
Negative Phrase: the deaf; deaf and dumb; suffers a hearing loss; afflicted with a hearing loss

Affirmative Phrase: person with a mental illness
Negative Phrase: crazy; psycho; lunatic

Affirmative Phrase: person with a developmental disability
Negative Phrase: retarded; mentally defective

Affirmative Phrase: person who uses a wheelchair
Negative Phrase: confined or restricted to a wheelchair; wheelchair bound

Affirmative Phrase: person with a physical disability; person with mobility impairment
Negative Phrase: cripple; lame; handicapped; deformed

Suggestions to Improve Access and Positive Interactions

• Avoid euphemisms such as 'physically challenged', 'special needs', 'differently abled' or 'handi-capped'. Many disability groups and individuals with disabilities object to these phrases because they are considered condescending and reinforce the idea that disabilities cannot be spoken of in an up front and direct manner.

• Do not sensationalise a disability by using terms such as 'afflicted with', 'suffers from', or 'crippled with'. These expressions are considered offensive and inaccurate to people with disabilities.

• When referring to people who use wheelchairs, avoid terms such as 'wheelchair bound' or 'confined to a wheelchair'. Wheelchairs do not confine people with disabilities; they provide freedom of movement and enable the user to travel more easily throughout the community.

• When writing or speaking about people with disabilities, emphasise abilities rather than limitations, focusing on a person's accomplishments, creative talents or skills. This does not mean avoiding mention of a person's disability, but doing so in a respectful manner. Here are some examples:

• When referring to a Guide Dog, do not call him a Blind Dog. Guide Dogs have great sight and they enable people with visual impairments and blindness to live independently.

Remember – if you are unsure about the proper way to refer to a person's disability, just ask the person about whom you are speaking or writing.

Interacting with People who are Visually Impaired or Blind

Don't
Shout when you speak to us, we can't see but our hearing is fine.

Do
Touch us on the arm or use our names when addressing us. This lets us know you are speaking to us, and not someone else in the room.

Don't
Grab us to lead us. Allow us to take your arm when we are walking together.

Do
Give specific directions like "the book is five feet to your right" as opposed to saying "the book is over there."

Don't
Pet or distract our Guide Dogs. They are not pets; they are working companions on whom we depend. Do not feed them anything as their health depends on a strict diet.

Do
Direct your questions directly to us. We do not need to have someone else tell us what we want to eat, etc.

Don't
Be afraid to use words like 'blind' or 'see'. Our eyes may not work but it is still nice to see you.

Do
Treat us as individuals. Blind people come in all shapes, sizes and colours. We each have our own strong points and weaknesses, just like everyone else.

Deafness and Communication

It is important to understand that for people who are deaf, **the major issue is not their inability to hear, but the challenges they experience in communicating with hearing people**. Speech develops as one imitates others and listens to the sounds they make, therefore vocal communication can be more complicated for people who have never heard speech than for those whose hearing loss developed later in life.

Many people who are deaf learn to use their voices in speech class and prefer to communicate vocally. Others choose to communicate in a variety of different ways, including sign language, speech reading (also known as *lip reading*), cued speech, and writing.

It is important to note that **sign language itself varies**. Irish Sign Language (iSL) is the most common form of sign language in Ireland. iSL is a full language with its own vocabulary, grammatical rules, and syntax that allows users to express themselves. It employs a subtle combination of hand, face, and body movements in communication. iSL is distinct from English and does not follow the word order, grammar rules, or syntax of the English language. iSL is not a universal sign language. People who are deaf from other countries may use other forms of sign language such as French sign language or Spanish sign language.

REMEMBER that shouting at a deaf person is of absolutely no benefit to them. Speak slowly and clearly. They will read your lips even if you do not make any vocal sound whilst speaking! Here are some tips to help you:

Do's and Don'ts In Communicating With a Deaf Person

Do
- Face the person
- Maintain good eye contact
- Speak slowly and clearly
- Have good light on your face
- Ask if you are being understood

Don't
- Shout
- Mutter
- Eat when speaking
- Smoke
- Obscure your mouth
- Turn your head away
- Give up

The smallest amount of effort will make life so much easier for you and the deaf person.

14. BLS and AED

When to Use a Defibrillator

"Around 270,000 people suffer a heart attack in the UK each year, about a third of whom die before reaching hospital due to cardiac arrest. A cardiac arrest most often occurs as a result of a heart attack, when the heart is starved of oxygen."

"Cardiac arrests cause the heart either to quiver, known as fibrillation or stop beating altogether. A defibrillator works by delivering a controlled electric shock through the chest wall to the heart to restore a normal heartbeat after a cardiac arrest."

British Heart Foundation press release, Friday 3 September 2004: *"2,300 new defibrillators to save lives across England."*

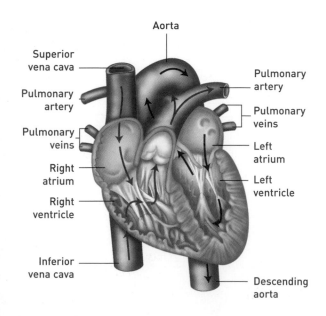

Figure 14.1: The heart.

The Heart Explained

The heart is a muscular pump, approximately the same size as its owner's fist, and is located behind and slightly to the left of the breastbone. Its function is to pump oxygen-rich blood from the lungs to various parts of the body, and to pump the de-oxygenated blood from the tissues back to the lungs to take on more oxygen. The heart pumps about 7,000 litres of blood around the body every day.

Pumping blood through the lungs removes carbon dioxide and re-supplies the blood with oxygen. The newly oxygenated blood is then pumped around the body to provide oxygen and nutrients and remove waste products.

The Heart's Mechanical Action

The heart has four chambers with one-way flaps called valves, between the upper and lower chambers. The atria are the upper chambers and they receive blood that is being returned to the heart. The right atrium receives blood with little oxygen in it because the blood has already circulated throughout the body delivering oxygen and nutrients. The left atrium fills with newly oxygenated blood returning from the lungs.

When the atria pump (contract), they push the blood through valves into the relaxed ventricles. When the ventricles contract, the right ventricle pumps blood into the lungs. The left ventricle pumps blood through the aortic valve to the body, including the heart (through coronary arteries). It is the pressure of the blood reflected on the walls of the arteries which is felt as a pulse.

A normal adult healthy heart beats rhythmically at a rate of about 60–100 beats per minute when at rest. During strenuous exercise, the heart can increase the amount of blood it pumps, up to four times the amount it pumps at rest, within only a matter of seconds. The source that drives this mechanical activity is *electrical stimulation*. This continuous cycle of synchronised contractions is driven by the heart's electrical system.

The Heart's Electrical System

The heart's electrical system causes the heart to beat, controls the heart rate (the number of beats per minute) and has special pathways (conduction pathways) that carry the electrical signals throughout the lower heart chambers (ventricles) for each heartbeat.

When heart cells in the upper heart chambers (atria) receive an electrical signal, they contract (pump) and then relax. The blood from the atria is pumped into the relaxed lower heart chambers (ventricles) and then pass down the separating tissue to the ventricles, causing them to contract and pump blood to the body.

On completion of the contraction of the ventricles, the electrical impulses cease, and the heart muscle relaxes.

Blood Circulation Cycle

Left Side of the Heart

The blood coming from the lungs to the heart collects in the left atrium, filling it up. The heart's electrical system sends a small electrical charge to the walls of the atria which initiates a contraction of the walls of the left atrium forcing the mitral valve to open as the blood gushes into the left ventricle.

The left ventricle fills with blood and an electrical signal initiates the muscle of the left ventricle to contract which forces the mitral valve to close, opens the aortic valve, and squeezes the blood through the aortic valve and into the body.

The blood coming out of the left ventricle to the aorta is under high pressure. This pressure is enough to rush it to the different parts of the body at high velocity and give its oxygen and nutrients to the body tissues. The blood comes back from the body to the right side of the heart.

Right Side of the Heart

The blood coming from the body to the heart collects in the right atrium, filling it up. The heart's electrical system sends a small electrical charge to the walls of the atria which initiates a contraction of the walls of the right atrium forcing the tricuspid valve to open as the blood gushes into the right ventricle.

The right ventricle fills with blood and an electrical signal initiates the muscle of the right ventricle to contract which forces the tricuspid valve to close, opens the pulmonary valve and squeeze the blood through the pulmonary valve and into the lungs. This blood will replenish itself with more oxygen and get rid of the carbon dioxide and return to the left side of the heart to begin another cycle.

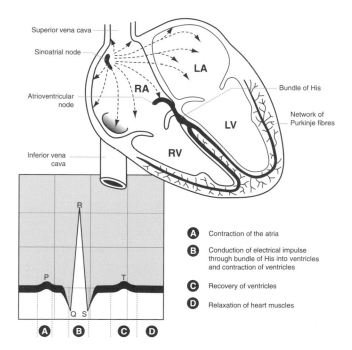

Figure 14.2: The electrical system of the heart.

The actions of the left side and right side of the heart occur simultaneously and are controlled by the electrical system of the heart. This electrical system generates a small electrical charge, which can be seen on a typical *ECG (electrocardiogram)* waveform (*see* figure 14.2).

The electrical system of the heart is made up of the following essential elements. The sinatrial (*SA) node* is the heart's "pacemaker" which generates a small electrical pulse at a rate of 60–100 pulses per minute at rest and increases this rate in response to the demands of the body for oxygen, for example during exercise or sporting activity. This initial small electrical pulse is seen on the ECG waveform as the *P wave* and it is this electrical signal which causes the muscles of the left and right atria to contract as described in the blood circulation cycle above.

As well as causing the atria to contract, this initial P wave is carried to the atrioventricular (*AV) node* which acts as a sort of electrical relay. The AV node delays the electrical pulse for a fraction of a second which can be seen as the small delay on the ECG waveform between the P wave and the Q wave. After this short delay, the AV node retransmits the electrical pulse to a network of conductive fibres called the *bundle of His* which sends the electrical signal to all parts of the left and right ventricles. The causes the muscles of the ventricles to contract strongly as described in the blood circulation cycle above. It is this strong contraction that is seen on the ECG waveform as the *QRS wave*. After this contraction has taken place the heart muscles relax and generate a small electrical signal, which is seen on the ECG wave as the T wave. The whole cycle then repeats at a rate of 60–100 cycles per minute (at rest) and can also be felt as the body's pulse. If you view the electrical waveform on a heart monitor or on an ECG recorder the normal rhythm will look something like this:

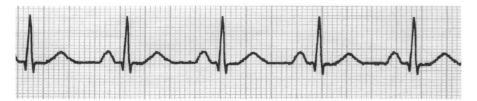

Figure 14.3: The electrical wave form on a heart monitor.

Understanding Sudden Cardiac Arrest and Defibrillation

What is Sudden Cardiac Arrest?

Sudden Cardiac Arrest (SCA) is one of the most common causes of death in developed countries. It is estimated that more than 3 million people worldwide die from SCA each year. SCA is an electrical malfunction of the heart typically associated with an abnormal heart rhythm known as *ventricular fibrillation (VF)*. It is a condition in which the heart's electrical impulses suddenly become chaotic, causing an abrupt cessation of the heart's pumping action. If you were able to view the electrical waveform of a patient suffering from ventricular fibrillation on a heart monitor or ECG recorder the rhythm will look something like this:

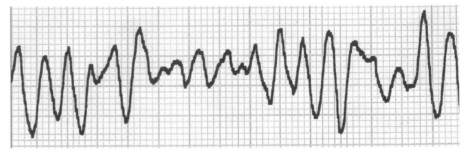

Figure 14.4: The electrical wave form of a patient suffering from ventricular fibrillation.

Victims collapse and quickly lose consciousness, often without warning. Unless a normal heart rhythm is restored, death follows within a matter of minutes. The average survival rate is less than five percent.

What Causes Sudden Cardiac Arrest?

SCA is largely unpredictable. Many victims have no prior history or symptoms of heart disease. One common cause, (but by no means the only cause) of sudden cardiac arrest is a heart attack (*myocardial infarction*). Heart attack is not strictly a recognised medical term. Most doctors prefer the term myocardial infarction or MI. A myocardial infarction occurs when you get a blockage in the small arteries that feed blood to the heart muscle itself. This usually results in the characteristic "crushing" chest pain felt by victims as the heart muscles are starved of oxygen. This oxygen starvation can sometimes trigger the chaotic heart rhythm called ventricular fibrillation described above, which causes the patient to collapse and have a sudden cardiac arrest. Sudden cardiac arrest can often occur in the early stages of a heart attack leading to collapse and death within a few minutes.

Other factors besides heart disease and heart attack can cause SCA, including respiratory arrest, electrocution, drowning, choking or trauma. In sports situations, SCA can sometimes be caused by physical impact on the chest over the heart (this has the medical term *commotio cordis*).

SCA in young apparently healthy adults or children can also be caused by undiagnosed problems with the heart which do not manifest themselves until the patient suffers an attack of SCA, frequently during a period of intense or sporting activity. In many cases, a fast and successful resuscitation attempt can provide enough time to allow the patient to be admitted to hospital to have the underlying cause of the arrest treated. Some people, for example those who have suffered a heart attack (myocardial infarction) in the past may be at higher risk.

How do I Recognise a Patient in Sudden Cardiac Arrest?

It can be very difficult to determine with certainty if a patient is suffering a sudden cardiac arrest. First you should determine if the patient is responsive to shouting and shaking (but be careful if physical injury is suspected especially to the neck or back). If the patient responds by moving or speaking or in any other way, they are probably not in cardiac arrest.

Secondly you should assess breathing. Look, listen and feel for any breathing. A patient breathing normally is probably not in cardiac arrest. Modern AED defibrillators are capable of very accurate analysis of a patient's heart rhythm. For this reason if you are in doubt about whether or not a patient is suffering from SCA, you should apply the defibrillator pads and let the defibrillator do the analysis. If the patient is responsive or breathing normally, you should not apply the defibrillator pads.

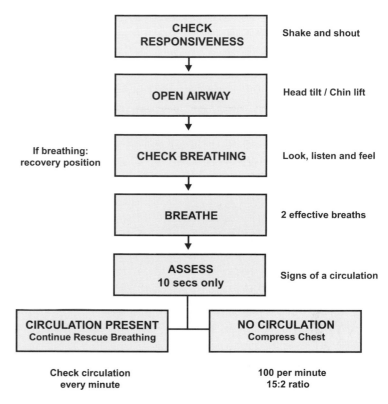

Figure 14.5: The UK Resuscitation Council guidelines offer this algorithm for basic life support.

The Role of the First Aider when SCA Occurs

The Chain of Survival

1st LINK – EARLY ACCESS
Call first – Call fast. Get to the cardiac arrest casualty quickly and call '999 or 112" for a cardiac ambulance.

2nd LINK – EARLY CPR
Early Cardiopulmonary Resuscitation (CPR) performed by a first aider on a patient who is in cardiac arrest can buy life-saving time.

3rd LINK – EARLY DEFIBRILLATION
Early defibrillation is the third and perhaps most significant link.

4th LINK – EARLY ACLS
Advanced Cardiac Life Support is provided by ambulance paramedics and other highly trained medical personnel.

How do you Treat Sudden Cardiac Arrest?

A heart in ventricular fibrillation must be defibrillated. To defibrillate the heart – to stop the chaotic and unproductive quivering of VF – an electrical shock must be applied. Defibrillation is recognized as the definitive treatment for ventricular fibrillation. Defibrillation administered within the first few minutes after collapse gives the patient the highest chance of survival. The likelihood of successful resuscitation decreases by approximately 7–10 percent with every minute that passes. After several minutes, very few resuscitation attempts are successful. Thus, the most important element in the treatment of SCA is providing rapid defibrillation therapy.

Does Early Defibrillation Guarantee Survival for the Patient?

Unfortunately there is no guarantee that early defibrillation will ensure a patient's resuscitation and survival. It may be impossible to restart the patient's heart for a number of reasons. Also a successful resuscitation is no guarantee of the long-term survival of the patient. Early defibrillation does however provide the best chance of resuscitation and survival for someone suffering sudden cardiac arrest. Defibrillation is the only treatment for sudden cardiac arrest due to fibrillation of the heart.

What is an Automated External Defibrillator (AED)?

An AED is a small, compact device that interprets heart rhythms and can deliver electrical shocks to treat sudden cardiac arrest.

The main difference between AEDs and the manually operated defibrillators often used by medical professionals is that AEDs are designed for use by people who may not have the extensive training required to use a manual defibrillator.

The new generation AEDs are very simple to operate. You don't need to recognize or interpret heart rhythms, because the AED does that automatically. One example is Philips HeartStart Home Defibrillator, which uses clear, natural voice instructions that guide the user through each step.

Is Defibrillation Hard to Learn?

Defibrillation (delivering an electrical shock to the heart) using an AED is easy to learn. The training takes just a short amount of time. For many people, operating an AED is easier to learn than CPR. Many fire fighters, first aid personnel, and flight attendants, as well as personnel in hospitals and clinics, have been performing manual defibrillation for years. More recently, flight attendants, first aid personnel, security staff, and others have used AEDs to help save lives. AEDs are being placed in medical and dental offices, clinics, health clubs, sports arenas, golf clubs, casinos, and other public places. Now with the introduction of the home Defibrillator, even ordinary people with no medical background can use an AED to help save a life.

Why the Need for "Early" Defibrillation?

Timing

Only one out of every 20 SCA victims survives – some of these lives could potentially be saved through timely defibrillation. With a brief window of opportunity for effective intervention, it is vital that a victim be defibrillated within the first few minutes of arresting. Published data also shows that nearly 80 percent of cardiac arrests occur in the home. Yet, survival rates are 30–50 percent lower than in public places with defibrillators. Because of this critical time factor, the first trained person at the patient's side should perform defibrillation. The American Heart Association and other national and international medical organizations are advocating defibrillation within five minutes of arrest.

Can AED Treatment Really Make a Difference?

It is a proven concept that the only effective treatment for SCA is prompt defibrillation. The availability of AED technology means that defibrillation can be a part of all CPR programs. When prompt defibrillation is combined with CPR, survival rates from sudden cardiac arrest dramatically improve.

The Case for Owning a Home Defibrillator

You should consult your GP or cardiologist before acquiring a home defibrillator for your own use. In the UK a prescription is NOT required to acquire a home defibrillator. A home defibrillator cannot be used by a person suffering a SCA on their own but can only be used by another person who witnesses the arrest and is willing and able to use the defibrillator. For this reason a home defibrillator is not usually suitable for use by people who live on their own. Anyone who is likely to use the defibrillator should be prepared to undertake some basic training and also be prepared to undergo some refresher self training at regular intervals. Basic training and self-training materials are provided by the AED supplier and certified training organisations.

The AED Unit for Home Use

The HeartStart home defibrillator is small, lightweight and easy-to-use. This unit is designed for use by members of the general public with minimal training. The battery-powered unit is ideal for the first aider to accompany their BLS skills to help save lives and also for any member of the public who may be faced with a situation of SCA in their homes, work or every day lives.

Using the AED Unit in Detail

The following instructions relate specifically to the Philips HeartStart Home Defibrillator, which has been cleared by the Food and Drug Administration (FDA) in the USA for sale to consumers 'over the counter' without a prescription. There are other defibrillators on the market and most work in a similar way. However, you should familiarise yourself with the operating procedures of any defibrillator you may be called upon to use.

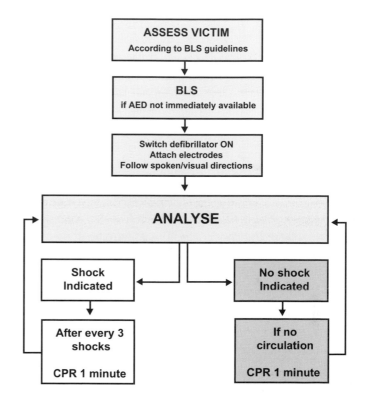

Figure 14.6: The UK Resuscitation Council published these guidelines for using an AED.

If you suspect you may have to use a defibrillator it is advisable to attend a short training course on the use of AEDs and to keep your training up-to-date. Choose a defibrillator that can be used by untrained users who simply follow the voice instructions. However, good quality training probably increases your chances of having a successful resuscitation when using an AED.

When preparing the victim for AED, remember the following important points. First, always check for your own safety. For example; if the patient has been electrocuted, you must ensure there is no risk to yourself before you approach the patient. Getting electrocuted yourself won't help the patient and just means that the next rescuer has TWO patients to deal with instead of one! Whatever the situation, it is important to assess your own safety and that of other bystanders before you proceed.

Using the guidelines of the RCUK (detailed above) you should next assess the patient. If you believe the patient is in cardiac arrest based on these guidelines, you should follow the BLS guidelines. If an AED is immediately at hand you should follow the AED guidelines. If an AED has to be located and brought to the scene, you should follow the BLS guidelines until the AED arrives at the scene and then follow the AED guidelines.

Remove all clothes from the chest area. This should be done with haste and not fumbling in an attempt to open buttons; "rip it, tear it, or cut it". If the patient's chest is wet (sweating is common) dry it quickly with a towel to help the pads stick correctly. If the patient has excess chest hair, clip or shave the area quickly to ensure good contact for the pads. You should also remove any medication patches and jewellery from the patient's chest area.

Pull the tab at the top of the pads cartridge off the film seal. Remove the pads (2 adhesive pads) from their liners. Place the pad on the chest as outlined in the picture on the pad itself. Press down firmly to secure the pads in place and repeat steps for the second pad. If for any reason the pads have lost their sticky quality and good contact is not made, remove and renew it immediately.

For Use on Children

For children up to 8 years of age, special child pads are required, and placement of these pads are different to an adult.

Once the pads are secured in place the unit will start analysing the rhythm of the patient's heart, and the caution light will start flashing. Once the unit commences operation, NO ONE must be in contact with the patient's body and the patient's body should not be moved.

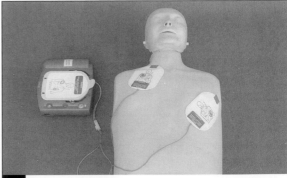
1. Place the pads.

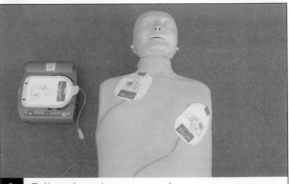
2. Follow the voice commands.

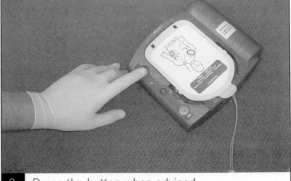
3. Press the button when advised.

If a Shock is Needed

The unit will take a few seconds to analyse the patient's heart rhythm. During this time the patient must not be touched and should not be moved. The defibrillator will advise you if a shock is needed and will instruct you to press the flashing orange shock button. Follow your clearance protocols and once it is safe, deliver the shock by pressing the flashing orange button. When the unit delivers the shock, the body may jerk suddenly. This is normal but make sure you are not so close that it comes in contact with you during the shock process. Once the shock has been delivered the unit will recommence analysing the rhythm of the heart and decide if another shock is required. If another shock is required, repeat the steps above. Once the shock button becomes live and a shock is required, you will have 30 seconds to press the button or the unit will disarm. The unit will constantly monitor the rhythm of the heart and if it changes (where a shock is no longer required) before you press the shock button, it will automatically disarm and advise you that a shock is not required.

Clearance Protocols

I AM CLEAR – assess that you are not in contact with the body.
YOU ARE CLEAR – assess that no bystanders are in contact with the body. Ask them to move back about 10 feet to minimise this risk.
WE ARE ALL CLEAR – a final check of this situation should be done before a shock is delivered.

By calling these steps out loud, it will assist you to clear people from the body, and if anything or anyone is touching the body they can shout to you. This will minimise the risk of the shock being delivered to that person also which would leave you with two patients instead of one.

If a Shock is not Required

If the unit analyses the heart rhythm and determines that a shock is not required, the blue light will come on and the unit will advise you that it is safe to touch the patient. Assess vital signs and commence BLS if required. During CPR, the unit may wish to analyse the heart rhythm and will instruct you to cease CPR.

On Arrival of the Ambulance

- Follow the guidance of the medical officers
- Advise them of your treatments
- Advise how long the patient has been down
- They may need to use a different defibrillator, so once instructed by them, remove your unit and pads
- They may also require data from your machine, so holding the "I" button down until it beeps will give them a spoken summary of the last use data
- It may be necessary for them to take this to the hospital with them
- Once you have briefed them, move to a safe distance and let them work
- Remain on site in case they need further information from you

Precautions

- Follow the instructions at all times
- Avoid air pocket formation under pads on the chest otherwise the patient may receive burns
- Always follow clearance protocols before shocking a patient
- Never use the unit near flammable gases
- Do not handle the unit aggressively
- Do not use the unit for any other reason than an emergency
- Only use the pads supplied by the manufacturer
- Pads required for small children and adults differ, so only use for the specific target group as provided
- During analysis of the heart rhythm, it is vital to minimise noise and movement around the body in order for the unit to get a clear reading. Electrical equipment or noise may disturb this process, so ask users of this equipment to turn them off
- Never operate in water or if the patient is lying in a pool of water

Appendix

Abbreviations

ACLS	Advanced Cardiac Life Support
AED	Automated External Defibrillator
BLS	Basic Life Support
CPR	Cardiopulmonary Resuscitation
CSF	Cerebrospinal Fluid
EMT	Emergency Medical Technician
FBAO	Foreign Body Airway Obstruction
LED	Light Emission Display
MI	Myocardial Infarction
NMT	Neuromuscular Therapy(ist)
SCA	Sudden Cardiac Arrest
TrP	Trigger Point(s)
VF	Ventricular Fibrillation

Anatomical Directions

ANTERIOR	in front of, or in the front part
POSTERIOR	behind, towards or in the back
DISTAL	situated away from the centre or midline of the body
PROXIMAL	nearest the trunk
INFERIOR	below in relation to some other structure
SUPERIOR	above in relation to some other structure
LATERAL	on or to the side, further from the midline
MEDIAL	relating to the middle or centre

FIRST AID ACCIDENT REPORT FORM

DATE	
TIME	
HISTORY OF ACCIDENT	
LOCATION	

FIRST AIDER'S NAME	
ADDRESS	
TELEPHONE	
PATIENT'S NAME	
ADDRESS	
TELEPHONE	
DATE OF BIRTH	
NEXT OF KIN	
ADDRESS	
TELEPHONE	
DOCTOR	
ADDRESS	
TELEPHONE	

INJURY DIAGNOSIS AND TREATMENT

INJURY 1 DIAGNOSIS	
TREATMENT GIVEN	
INJURY 2 DIAGNOSIS	
TREATMENT GIVEN	
INJURY 3 DIAGNOSIS	
TREATMENT GIVEN	

INJURY DIAGNOSIS AND TREATMENT

PULSE	RESPIRATION	TEMPERATURE
1.		
2.		
3.		

MEDICAL HISTORY

ALLERGIES	CURRENT MEDICATIONS

MEDICAL HISTORY

DOCTOR OR AMBULANCE OFFICER	
ADDRESS	
TELEPHONE	

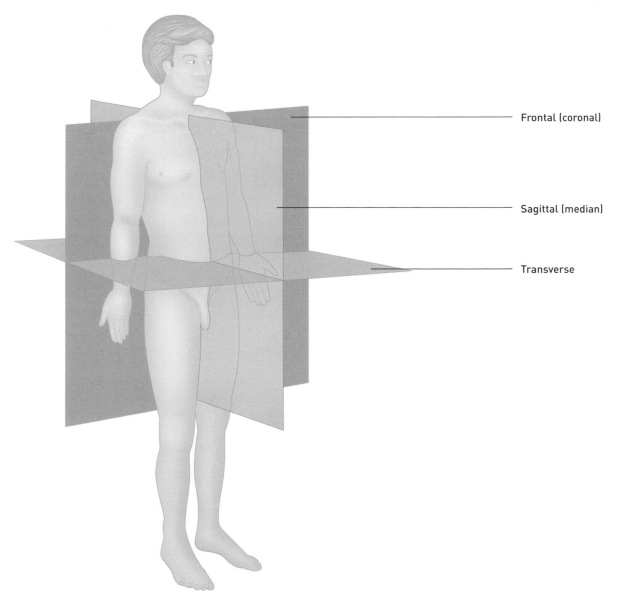

Frontal (coronal)

Sagittal (median)

Transverse

Figure A1: Planes of the body.

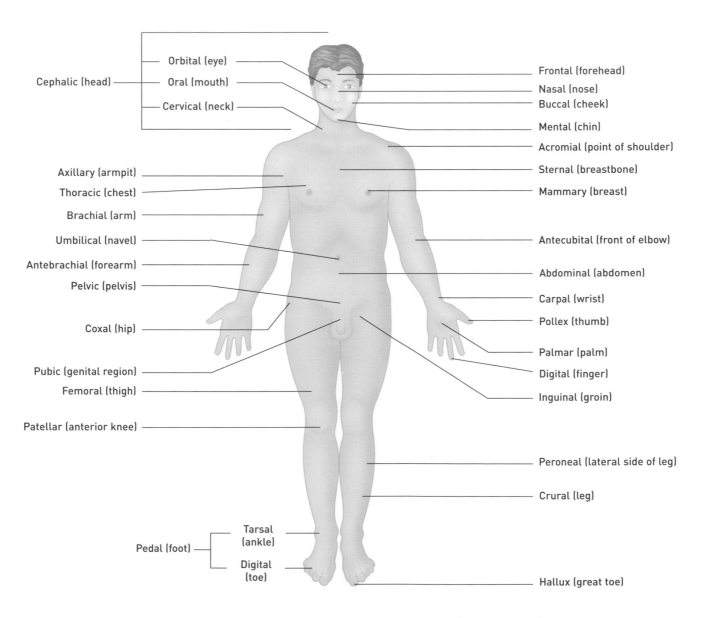

Cephalic (head)
Orbital (eye)
Oral (mouth)
Cervical (neck)

Frontal (forehead)
Nasal (nose)
Buccal (cheek)
Mental (chin)
Acromial (point of shoulder)
Sternal (breastbone)
Mammary (breast)

Axillary (armpit)
Thoracic (chest)
Brachial (arm)
Umbilical (navel)
Antebrachial (forearm)
Pelvic (pelvis)
Coxal (hip)
Pubic (genital region)
Femoral (thigh)
Patellar (anterior knee)

Antecubital (front of elbow)
Abdominal (abdomen)
Carpal (wrist)
Pollex (thumb)
Palmar (palm)
Digital (finger)
Inguinal (groin)

Peroneal (lateral side of leg)
Crural (leg)

Pedal (foot)
Tarsal (ankle)
Digital (toe)
Hallux (great toe)

Figure A2: Terms used to indicate specific body areas (anterior view).

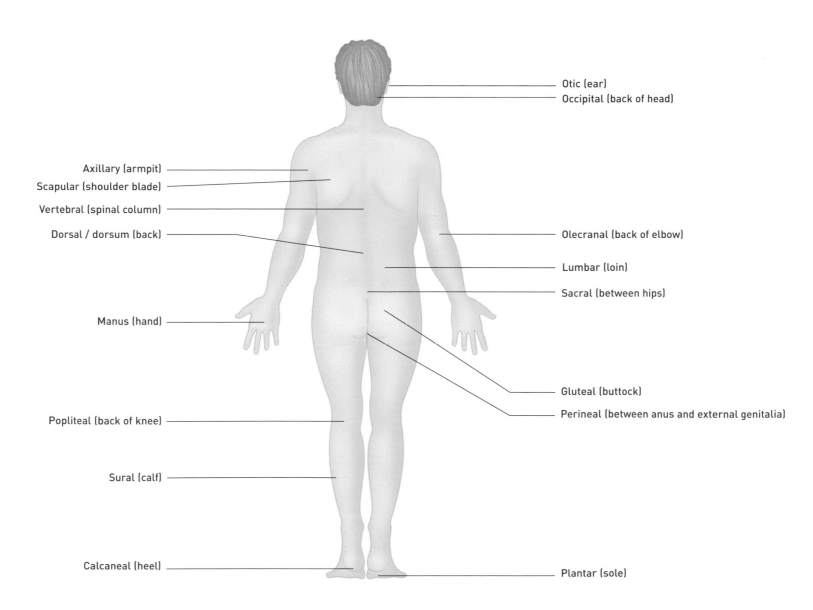

Otic (ear)
Occipital (back of head)

Axillary (armpit)
Scapular (shoulder blade)
Vertebral (spinal column)
Dorsal / dorsum (back)

Olecranal (back of elbow)

Lumbar (loin)

Sacral (between hips)

Manus (hand)

Gluteal (buttock)

Perineal (between anus and external genitalia)

Popliteal (back of knee)

Sural (calf)

Calcaneal (heel)

Plantar (sole)

Figure A3: Terms used to indicate specific body areas (posterior view).

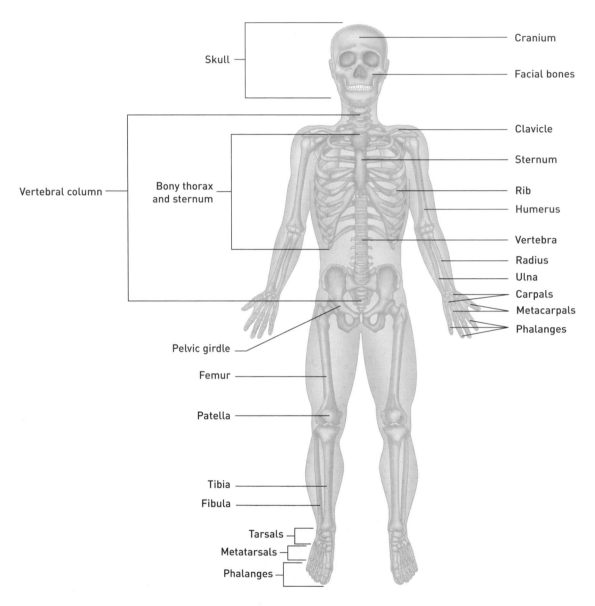

Skull
— Cranium
— Facial bones

Vertebral column

Bony thorax and sternum
— Clavicle
— Sternum
— Rib
— Humerus
— Vertebra
— Radius
— Ulna
— Carpals
— Metacarpals
— Phalanges

Pelvic girdle

Femur

Patella

Tibia
Fibula

Tarsals
Metatarsals
Phalanges

Figure A4: The skeletal system (anterior view).

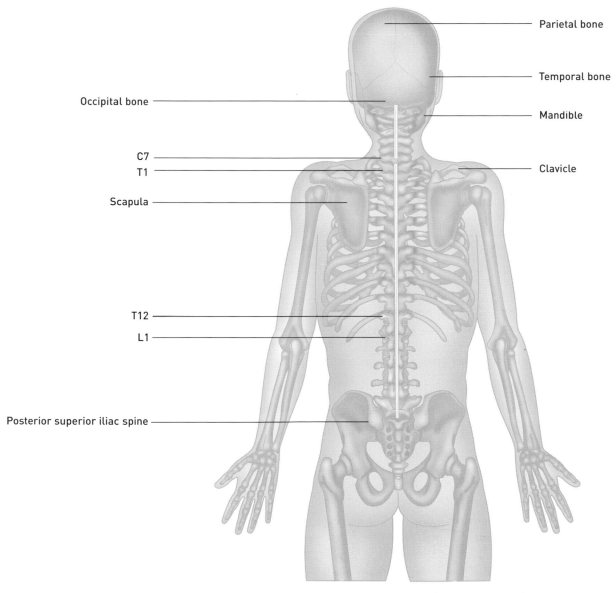

Parietal bone

Temporal bone

Occipital bone

Mandible

C7

T1

Clavicle

Scapula

T12

L1

Posterior superior iliac spine

Figure A5: The skeletal system (posterior view).

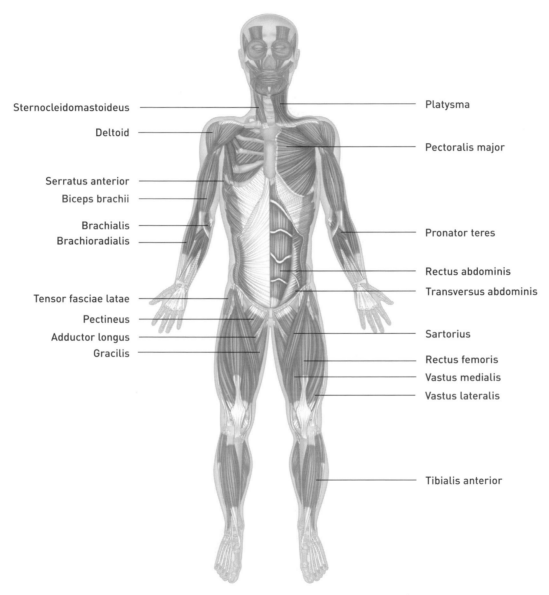

Sternocleidomastoideus

Deltoid

Serratus anterior

Biceps brachii

Brachialis

Brachioradialis

Tensor fasciae latae

Pectineus

Adductor longus

Gracilis

Platysma

Pectoralis major

Pronator teres

Rectus abdominis

Transversus abdominis

Sartorius

Rectus femoris

Vastus medialis

Vastus lateralis

Tibialis anterior

Figure A6: The muscular system (anterior view).

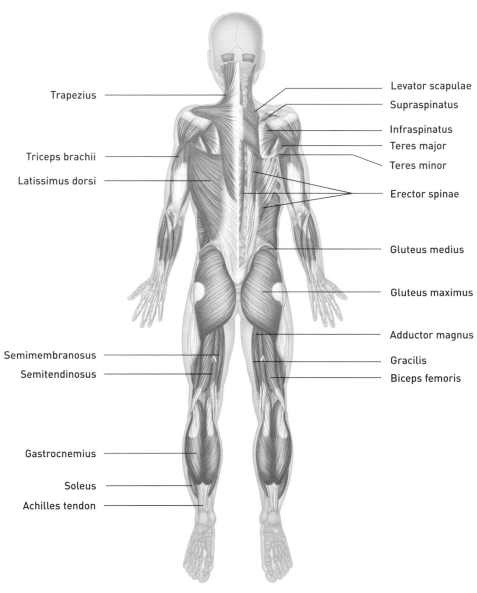

Trapezius

Triceps brachii

Latissimus dorsi

Semimembranosus

Semitendinosus

Gastrocnemius

Soleus

Achilles tendon

Levator scapulae

Supraspinatus

Infraspinatus

Teres major

Teres minor

Erector spinae

Gluteus medius

Gluteus maximus

Adductor magnus

Gracilis

Biceps femoris

Figure A7: The muscular system (posterior view).

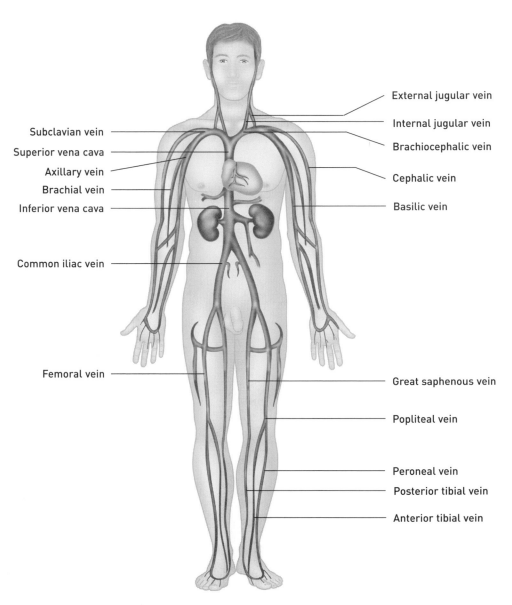

Figure A8: A general overview of major veins and branches.

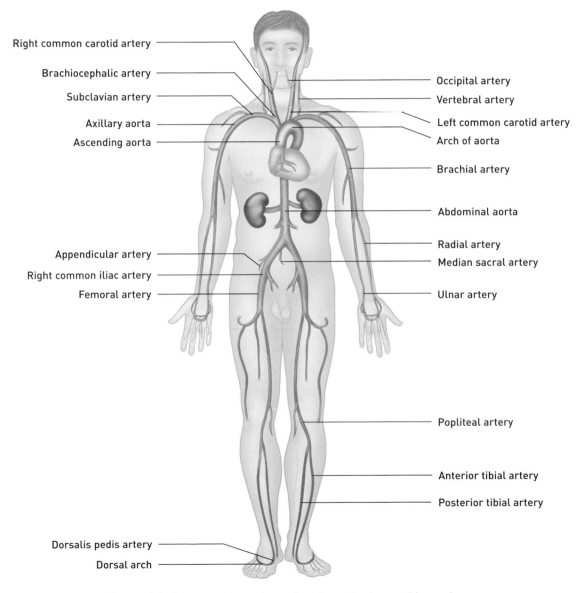

Right common carotid artery

Brachiocephalic artery

Subclavian artery

Axillary aorta

Ascending aorta

Occipital artery

Vertebral artery

Left common carotid artery

Arch of aorta

Brachial artery

Abdominal aorta

Radial artery

Median sacral artery

Appendicular artery

Right common iliac artery

Femoral artery

Ulnar artery

Popliteal artery

Anterior tibial artery

Posterior tibial artery

Dorsalis pedis artery

Dorsal arch

Figure A9: A general overview of major arteries and branches.

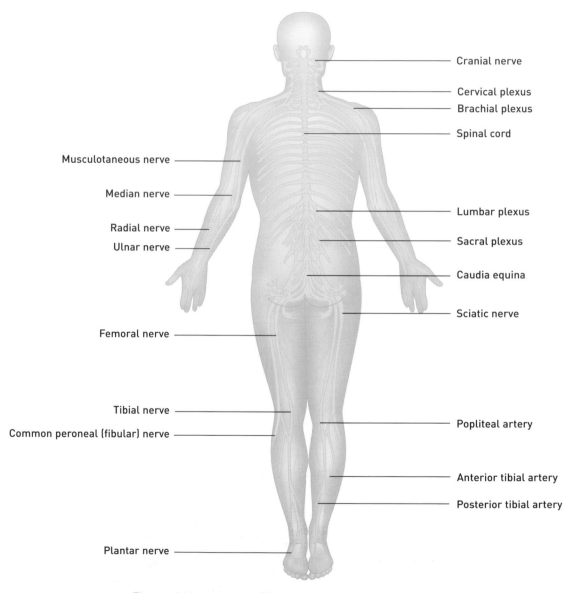

Cranial nerve

Cervical plexus

Brachial plexus

Spinal cord

Musculotaneous nerve

Median nerve

Lumbar plexus

Radial nerve

Sacral plexus

Ulnar nerve

Caudia equina

Sciatic nerve

Femoral nerve

Tibial nerve

Popliteal artery

Common peroneal (fibular) nerve

Anterior tibial artery

Posterior tibial artery

Plantar nerve

Figure A10: A general overview of major peripheral nerves.

Useful Addresses

Training Establishments

Direct First Aid
82. The Spinney, Beaconsfield
Buckinghamshire, HP9 1SA, UK
Tel.: 44 (0) 1494 678221 / 44 (0) 1494 764666
Fax.: 44 (0) 1494 681284
E-mail: info@directfirstaid.biz
www.directfirstaid.biz

D-Stress Direct (UK), Corporate Therapies
Tel.: 44 (0) 1494 764666
e-mail: info@d-stressdirect.biz
www.d-stressdirect.biz

F.A.S.T., First Aid and Sports Therapy
12. Beal Srutha, Ballybane, Galway, Ireland
Tel.: 00 (353 8) 74163726
e-mail: fastgalway@hotmail.com

Federation of Holistic Therapists
3rd Floor, Eastleigh House, Upper Market Street
Eastleigh, SO50 9FD, UK
Tel.: 44 (0) 23 8048 8950
Fax.: 44 (0) 23 8048 8970
E-mail: info@fht.org.uk

For more information on Neuromuscular Therapy (NMT) or to locate a professional NMT / Physical Therapist in your geographical location contact:

National Training Centre
16a. Saint Joseph's Parade, Dorset Street, Dublin 7, Ireland
Tel.: 00 (353 1) 8827777.   London office: 08000 851094
Fax.: 00 (353 1) 8308757
e-mail: neuromusculartherapy@ntc.ie
www.ntc.ie

Judith DeLany, NMT Center
900 14th Avenue North, St. Petersburg, Florida 33705, USA
Tel.: 00 (1) 727 821 7167
Fax.: 00 (1) 727 822 0643

Practitioner Training and Development Associates
Tel.: 44 (0) 1494 764666 or 44 (0) 1494 678221
e-mail: info@acupressure-training.co.uk
www.acupressure-training.co.uk

Resuscitation Council (UK)
5th Floor, Tavistock House North, Tavistock Square
London, WC1H 9HR, UK
Tel.: 44 (0) 20 73884678
e-mail: enquiries@resus.org.uk
www.resus.org.uk

Suppliers

Brompton Home Health Ltd.
Sole UK distributor of Philips HeartStart Home Defibrillator
54. Market Street, Whaley Bridge, High Peak
Derbyshire, SK23 7AA, UK
Tel.: 44 (0) 1663 732587
Fax.: 44 (0) 1633 719366
e-mail: carr@medintellect.com
www.brompton.net

Forsport Ltd., supplier of goods to football
2. Brook Court, 3. Blakeney Road
Beckenham, Kent, BR3 1HG, UK
Tel.: 44 (0) 20 8658 2007 (Forsport UK)
Tel.: 44 (0) 20 8650 0022 (Forsport Europe)
Fax.: 44 (0) 20 8658 1314
e-mail: info@forsport.co.uk
www.forsport.co.uk

Heath Affairs Ltd., UK distributor of CPREzy
Unit 1, Claremont Way Industrial Estate
London, NW2 1AL, UK
Tel.: 44 (0) 20 8905 5999
Fax.: 44 (0) 20 8905 5222
e-mail: info@healthaffairs.co.uk
www.healthaffairs.co.uk

Houghton's Books, supplier of books
Topshill, Kirk Ireton, Derbyshire, DE6 3JX, UK
Tel.: 44 (0) 7980 775223
Fax.: 44 (0) 1629 822272

L+M First Aid Medical, supplier of First Aid Kits
Registered office: Kilkerrin
Ballinasloe, Co. Galway, Ireland
Tel. 00 (353 9) 345685; 00 (353 9) 345684

MDAL, CPREzy supplier in Ireland
73. Admiral Park
Baldoyle
Dublin 13
Tel: 00 (353 8) 7232 0346

Seaberg Company, supplier of the SAM® Splint
4909 S. Coast Highway, Suite 245
Newport, Oregon 97365, USA
Tel.: 00 (1) 541 867 4726
Fax.: 00 (1) 541 867 4646
Toll Free 800 818 4726
e-mail: info@samsplint.com

SP Services (UK) Ltd., supplier of First Aid equipment
Unit D4, Hortonpark Estate, Hortonwood 7
Telford, Shropshire, TF1 7GX, UK
Tel.: 44 (0) 1952 288970
Fax.: 44 (0) 1952 288987
e-mail: info@spservices.co.uk
www.spservices.co.uk

Index

Achilles tendon strain 80
Alveoli 30
Anaphylaxis 105
Angina 31
Anterior compartment pain 79
Appendicular skeleton 51
Arm bones 51
Arteries 25, 139
  coronary 120
Asthma 102
Athlete's foot 79
Atrioventricular (AV) node 122
Atrium 120
Automated external defibrillator (AED) 123
Axial skeleton 48

Biomechanical dysfunction 74
Black eyes 110
Bleeding 25
  external 27
  internal 27
Blood circulation cycle 121
Blood loss control 26
Blood vessels 25
Body check 19
Bony thorax 50
Brain 88
Breathing 19
Broken tooth 111
Bronchi 30
Bundle of His 122

Calcification 53
Capillaries 25
Capillary refill 19
Cardiac arrest 32
Cardiopulmonary resuscitation (CPR)
  adult 32
  child 34
Carpal tunnel syndrome 81
Chest wound, penetrating 96
Circulatory system 24
Closed wound 26
Cold therapy 75
Coma 89
Compression 84
Connective tissue sheath 76
CPRezy 43
Cramp 78
Cranial bones 48

Deafness 118
Defibrillator 120
Diabetes 103
Diaphragm 30
Dislocation 77
Distraction 84
Drug poisoning 101
Duramater 88

Ear injuries 112
Electrical stimulation 120
Electrocardiogram (ECG) 122
Epilepsy 104
Eye abrasions 110

Facial bones 49
Fainting 98
First aid room 15
Flail chest 95
Foreign body airway obstruction (FBA)
  adult 36, 37
  child 38, 39
Fractures 53
  causes 54
  types 53
Friction burns 113
Frostbite 107
Frostnip 107

Golfer's elbow 81

Heart 31, 120
Heart attack 30, 32, 122
Heat exhaustion 99
Heat stroke 100
Heat therapy 75
Heel spurs 79
Hepatitis B Virus (HBV) 25
Human Immuno-deficiency Virus (HIV) 25
Hyperextension 84
Hyperflexion 84
Hyperglycaemia 103
Hypoglycaemia 103

Ice therapy, *see* cold therapy
Immunoglobulin E (IgE) 105
Infection control 26

Inflammation	74
Ischemia	74
Jaw thrust	42
Lateral flexion	84
Leg bones	52
Ligaments	76
Lip reading	118
Log roll	86
Medical history, patient's	21, 30
Metatarsalgia	78
Muscular system	136, 137
Myocardial infarction, *see* heart attack	
Nerve compression	74
Nerves, peripheral	140
Neuromuscular therapy	74
Nose bleeds	110
Open airway	42
Open wound	26
Pectoral girdle	51
Pelvic girdle	52
People-first	116
Planes of the body	131
Poisoning	100
Posterior compartment pain	80
Postural distortion	74
Pre-event checklist	16
Prevention tips	81
Primary survey	18
Pulse	19
Recovery position	40
Repetitive strain injury (RSI)	78
Respiration	30
Ribcage	94

Rib,	
false	94
floating	94
fractured	94
true	94
SAMPLE scale	21
Secondary survey	18
Shin splints	80
Shock	21
Sinoatrial (SA) node	122
Skeletal muscle	76
Skeletal system	134, 135
Skin condition	19
Skull	48
Snake bites	101
Soft tissue injuries, prevention of	75
Sports first aid kit	14
Sprains	76
State of stupor	89
Strains	77
Sudden cardiac arrest (SCA)	122
Sunburn	99
Tendons	76
Tennis elbow	80
Thomas half-ring splint	71
Tooth dislodgement	111
Trigger points	74
Unconsciousness	89
Valves	120
Veins	25, 138
Ventricle	121
Ventricular fibrillation (VF)	122
Verbal stimuli	89
Vertebra	50
Vertebral column	84
Visually impaired	117

Wounds	26, 27